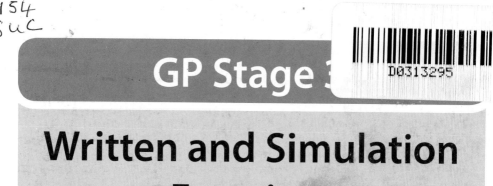

# GP Stage 3

## Written and Simulation Exercises

# GP Stage 3:

# Written and Simulation Exercises

**Richard Hughes** BMedSci BMBS MRCS nMRCGP DPD

General Practitioner, Kingston Health Centre, Kingston upon Thames
United Kingdom

**Shivani Tanna** BSc MBBS nMRCGP DRCOG

General Practitioner, Millbank Medical Centre, London
United Kingdom

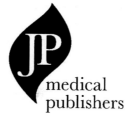

JP
medical
publishers

London • St Louis • Panama City • New Delhi

© 2013 JP Medical Ltd.
Published by JP Medical Ltd
83 Victoria Street, London, SW1H 0HW, UK
Tel: +44 (0)20 3170 8910       Fax: +44 (0)20 3008 6180
Email: info@jpmedpub.com       Web: www.jpmedpub.com

ISBN: 978-1-907816-61-1

**British Library Cataloguing in Publication Data**
A catalogue record for this book is available from the British Library

**Library of Congress Cataloging in Publication Data**
A catalog record for this book is available from the Library of Congress

JP Medical Ltd is a subsidiary of Jaypee Brothers Medical Publishers (P) Ltd, New Delhi, India

| | |
|---|---|
| Publisher: | Richard Furn |
| Senior Editorial Assistant: | Katrina Rimmer |
| Design: | Designers Collective Ltd |

Typeset, printed and bound in India.

# Preface

The GP Stage 3 Selection Centre process was introduced in 2007. It has evolved over the years into an excellent way of selecting candidates who have the attributes to become good general practitioners. In 2011 the process was amended and it now includes three consultation tasks and a written exercise (the old group exercise discussed in other revision guides no longer exists).

Applications to train in general practice have increased over the past few years and so the selection process, especially for the most popular deaneries, has become extremely competitive. However, there is no doubt that focussed practice improves candidate performance and, with this level of competition, being well prepared is vitally important. Practice and preparation may be the difference between getting a job or not, or getting your first choice rotation rather than your tenth.

This book has been written to help you get through the selection process. As well as discussing how to approach written prioritisation exercises and simulated consulatations, it is based on cases and concepts that have arisen over the last few years at selection centres. It focuses on the areas candidates find difficult and includes 60 practice exercises. We often find that people attending our course are keen to note down key phrases and find our own example answers and consultation videos very useful. For this reason, this book provides 15 examples of completed written exercises and 45 transcribed consultations highlighting the different communication techniques discussed in the preceding chapters.

Richard Hughes
Shivani Tanna
November 2012

# Contents

# GP Stage 3 Selection Centre: the application process

## The application process has three stages:

**Stage 1:** Demonstrating and assessing eligibility via an online application form

**Stage 2:** Written examination

- Paper 1: professional dilemmas and situational judgement
- Paper 2: clinical problem solving

**Stage 3:** Selection centre

- Simulation exercises: three 10-minute simulated exercises
  1. Consultation with a patient
  2. Consultation with a relative or carer
  3. Consultation with a non-medical colleague
- Written exercise: 30 minutes in which to rank or prioritise issues with written justification for your responses

Your regional allocation to a selection centre will depend on your score at stage 2, and the final allocation of jobs within each deanery will depend on your performance at both stage 2 and stage 3.

## How to use this book

We recommend that you do all of the written exercises under strict exam conditions, giving yourself 30 minutes per case. After this, read your answers back and reflect on whether you have:

1. Written legibly with answers that are clear to understand
2. Understood the issues raised in the case
3. Prioritised sensibly
4. Justified your decisions
5. Described the actions you would take
6. Utilised the different team members appropriately
7. Demonstrated some of the attributes of a good GP (outlined in Chapter 1)
8. Left enough time to complete the task

The simulated consultation exercises are best worked through in groups of three people: one can be the candidate, one the actor and one the examiner. It is important to be strict with timings and stop the case after 10 minutes so that you get a feel for what the time pressure will be like on the day. On completion of each case it important to get feedback from your peers and ask yourself the following:

1. Did I establish a good rapport?
2. Did I ask open questions?
3. Did I allow the patient to speak?
4. Did I gather all the relevant information and get to the bottom of the problem?
5. Was my consultation well structured?

While we do not propose that you read all of the transcripts, we encourage you to use them as a resource if you found a case difficult, are wondering how specific situations could be approached or are looking for succinct phrases to help your own consultations.

## How to prepare for the assessment

Try to attend a course before you do your selection centre. Be sure to research the courses before booking. A good course will allow you to practice every element of the Stage 3 process with small group work and individual feedback from experienced tutors (not feedback provided by other candidates) who will quickly be able to focus in on your own learning needs.

# What to remember on the day of your selection centre

Arrive on time and make sure you are fully aware of where the selection centre is being held. Long journeys should be planned in advance and you should expect to be there for half a day (morning or afternoon).

Take all the paperwork you are required to present on the day as stated by your deanery. This usually includes:

1. Passport or driving licence
2. Your original medical qualification certificate
3. Original evidence of foundation competencies
4. Hard copies of your structured reference forms if your referees have not submitted them online
5. Photocopies of the above

It is recommended that you wear smart clothing that you would wear on a day-to-day basis when expecting to deal with patients. If in doubt, dress slightly more smartly than you would normally. Things to avoid are:

- Any revealing clothing (short skirts, low-cut tops)
- Dangling jewellery
- Inappropriate hair styles with untied long hair
- Any form of dress covering the face

If you feel you should be eligible for extra time in the written examination or the written element, due to a proven condition such as dyslexia, then this should be requested from the recruitment office well in advance, during the application process.

Good luck on the day and remember to remain calm. If you feel one exercise has gone badly it is important to clear your head and move onto the next assessment. Remember each exercise is marked independently and very few candidates feel that the whole process went perfectly.

# Acknowledgements

We would like to thank the following people for their contribution to the preparation of this book:

Denula Suthaharan

Neha Kataria

Anna Humphries

Amit Patel

Sally Hughes

Andrew Hughes

Rekha Tanna

Suresh Tanna

# Glossary

| | |
|---|---|
| **A&E** | Accident and emergency |
| **ABC** | Airway, breathing, circulation |
| **Anti-CCP** | Anti-citrullinated protein |
| **CLO** | *Campylobacter*-like organism |
| **COPD** | Chronic obstructive pulmonary disease |
| **CPD** | Continuing professional development |
| **CT** | Computed tomography |
| **CTPA** | CT pulmonary angiogram |
| **DIY** | Do-it-yourself |
| **DOB** | Date of birth |
| **DOPS** | Directly observed procedural skills |
| **DVT** | Deep vein thrombosis |
| **ECG** | Electrocardiography |
| **ICE** | Ideas, concerns and expectations |
| **FBC** | Full blood count |
| **FY1** | Foundation year 1 |
| **FY2** | Foundation year 2 |
| **GMC** | General Medical Council |
| **GP** | General practitioner |
| **GUM** | Genitourinary medicine |
| **HCA** | Healthcare assistant |
| **HIV** | Human immunodeficiency virus |
| **INR** | International normalised ratio |
| **ID** | Identification |
| **IT** | Information technology |
| **ITU** | Intensive treatment unit |
| **MDT** | Multidisciplinary team |
| **MRI** | Magnetic resonance imaging |
| **MRSA** | Methicillin-resistant *Staphylococcus aureus* |
| **MS** | Multiple sclerosis |
| **NSTEMI** | Non-ST elevation myocardial infarction |
| **OPA** | Outpatient appointment |
| **PALS** | Patient advice and liaison service |
| **RA** | Rheumatoid arthritis |
| **SHO** | Senior house officer |
| **TTO** | To take out |

# Chapter 1

# Written prioritisation exercises: introduction

## Introduction

The written prioritisation exercise is an extremely time-pressured 30-minute task. At first glance it seems simple enough but scoring highly requires thought and preparation. This chapter outlines exactly what the task involves and what you will need to do to score highly.

As you work through this chapter and the subsequent worked examples you'll notice that certain themes are repeated time after time. Candidates often find that they can incorporate well-structured fluent phrases from earlier practised examples into their answers on the day itself.

Try to complete as many of the examples as you can under exam conditions, then review your answers and think about how they could be improved. Chapter 2 provides example answers to all of the exercises to give you an idea of how to demonstrate the various attributes required to score highly, but we encourage you to bring out your own individuality into your answers.

## The written prioritisation exercise

You will have 30 minutes in which five tasks have to be prioritised. You are expected to write a justification for each priority, explaining your reasons for ordering each in your chosen way, and then describe practical actions you would take to complete the task.

You will be given instructions explaining what your role is. This is usually a doctor at the level of foundation year two in a hospital, or less commonly in a primary care setting. You will be told that you have a limited time period in which to complete five different tasks. For example:

> You are an FY2 doctor working on an orthopaedic ward. You have to leave in 1 hour to catch a flight to go on holiday. The following tasks are pending and require your attention.
>
> A. The ward clerk has called you to bring some notes you were using that you have left in the doctor's office.
> B. One of the nurses calls you to write up fluids for a postoperative patient who has low blood pressure.
> C. Your consultant has arranged to meet you to do your end of placement clinical supervisor review.

      D. The relatives of a patient who has come out of theatre following
         a fractured neck of femur repair have asked to speak with you.

      E. Your FY1 has called you as she is unable to insert a cannula on
         a patient and needs some help.

Initially you have to rank these in the order in which you would prioritise them using letters (A–E) or numbers (1–5). For each task you will have a paragraph in which to write your answer that should include the following in each box:

- Which priority?
- Why you prioritised it in this way?
- How you would go about completing the task?

In addition you will be asked to reflect on the task. This most commonly involves answering three separate questions. For example:

1. What did you find difficult when completing this task?
2. What did you learn about yourself during this task?
3. What you would do differently if you could do this task again?

The worked examples in this book use this format in the reflection, but do expect to find some variations on the day. For example:

1. What did you find easy during this task and why?
2. What are the limitations of this task?
3. How would you approach this differently if you were asked to repeat the exercise?

GP selection is designed for doctors with at least 18 months of clinical experience and so this exercise will involve tasks that are feasible for you to encounter in your jobs as a junior doctor. It is not supposed to be a test of your clinical acumen but rather your ability to organise your time, work efficiently as part of a team, recognise situations where there is clinical risk and solve problems.

You are expected to write your answers in full sentences, avoiding the use of bullet points, and you should aim to demonstrate good written communication with clear, articulate use of language.

The exercises are marked by experienced general practitioners who will be looking for you to demonstrate some of the attributes required to work effectively in primary care. Some of the most important of these can be remembered using a simple mnemonic, **DOTT: Delegation, Organisation, Time management, Team work.**

## Teamwork

Make sure you use other members of the team to help you complete the tasks – this demonstrates that you are realistic and appreciate the value of your colleagues. You are NOT expected to complete all of the tasks by yourself; recognising your own capabilities and limitations within the restricted time period is something you should try to demonstrate in your answers.

**Table 1.1** outlines the members of staff available in different medical settings. You may be able to draw upon some of these to help you achieve all of the tasks efficiently.

## Table 1.1 Members of primary care and hospital teams

| Primary care team members | Hospital team members |
| --- | --- |
| Receptionists | FY1 doctors |
| Secretaries | Registrars |
| Read coders | Consultants |
| Health visitors | Phlebotomists |
| Physiotherapists | Healthcare assistants |
| Counsellors | Physiotherapists |
| Salaried GPs | Ward clerks |
| GP partners | Porters |
| Health visitors | Secretaries |
| Social workers | Occupational therapists |
| District nurses | Speech and language therapists |
| Phlebotomists | Discharge coordinators |
| Healthcare assistants | Nurses |
| Practice managers | Interpreters |
| Community pharmacists | Pharmacists |
| Osteopaths | Dieticians |
| | Security guards |
| | Human resources and administrative staff |

## The person specification

The GP recruitment process was designed to select the candidates that best match against the personal attributes required to be a good GP. Think about the skills and attributes listed below and try to demonstrate them in your answers.

- Empathy and sensitivity.
- Communication skills.
- Clinical knowledge and expertise.
- Conceptual thinking and problem solving.
- Personal organisational and administrative skills.
- Professional integrity.
- Coping with pressure.
- Managing stress and team involvement.
- Legal, ethical and political awareness.

### Empathy and sensitivity

Empathy and sensitivity are difficult to demonstrate in a written exercise but with deeper thought into the tasks presented, and the wider implications of some of these, it can easily be achieved. For example, if a case involves talking to the bereaved family of patient, explaining that you would not want to keep them waiting as you recognise what a difficult time this must be for them, and offering an apology for any delay incurred, will certainly demonstrate both empathy and sensitivity.

This may seem easy to do with an emotive situation like this one. However, even with a simpler task, such as having to meet your consultant to carry out an assessment, it is possible to demonstrate empathy and sensitivity by stating that it is important to try to rearrange this at the earliest opportunity because your consultant is also very busy and you do not want to waste his/her time.

### Clinical knowledge and expertise

Specific clinical knowledge has already been tested during your written examinations but during the written exercise you would be expected to show awareness of the clinical importance of certain situations and potential consequences of each. Patient safety should always be of paramount importance and this should be reflected in your answers. Decisiveness is also an important skill to portray.

### Conceptual thinking and problem solving

Problem solving requires you to think laterally and adopt a sensible and pragmatic approach. The solutions you consider should be realistic and in some cases creative. Writing clearly and concisely can show that you are systematic especially if your answers are well structured. Certain tasks will be purposely ambiguous so try to recognise this and acknowledge it in your answer. This shows the ability to think analytically with a deeper understanding of the issues.

### Professional integrity

Demonstrating professional integrity is important. You should try to show that you are willing to take responsibility for your own actions and respect your colleagues.

Recognising the wider implications of certain issues and your actions, and stating these, can make your approach appear more sophisticated and professional. For example, if a medication error has occurred one could go a step further and talk about filling out an incident form for the matter to be investigated further, in order to learn from it and prevent the mistake occurring in the future.

Continual professional development (CPD) is vital for all doctors. Commonly tasks arise that involve CPD, e.g. completing application forms, learning new procedures, appraisal meetings. It may be necessary to postpone or delay these, but you should make a point of recognising their importance.

Legal or ethical implications need to be considered carefully. Even if you are uncertain what to do this can be reflected on to at least show that these issues have been considered.

## Allocation of time

The tasks will vary from clinical emergencies to seemingly trivial tasks such as paying a cheque into the bank before it closes. Some tasks will seem less important than others but an equal amount of time and emphasis should be dedicated to each, as there are marks to be gained from every section. It is therefore important to manage your time in order to complete each section, including your reflection.

For effective time management you will need to practise as many of these exercises as possible. Once you have decided which order you want to prioritise the tasks in, there is very little time to change your answers half way through – it's more important to complete the exercise. You will have the opportunity to state that you may have done things in a different order and your reasons for this later on in the reflection.

A suggested framework to guide your time management:

- 3 minutes to read the scenarios and gather your thoughts.
- 4 minutes to rank each issue and write your justification and action.
- 6 minutes to write your reflection on the task.

## GMC duties of a doctor

The basis for good and safe clinical practice is outlined by the GMC guidance (see reference, p. 7). This guidance forms the basis on which the written prioritisation exercise is marked. Applying these principles in your answers will show good understanding of good practice as a doctor. There are areas in this guidance on which you should focus:

- Ensuring patient safety and care is your main concern.
- Health promotion.
- Providing a good standard of care by maintaining personal and professional development, recognising limitations and working within your own competence level, and working well with colleagues.
- Respecting colleagues and patients and maintaining confidentiality.
- Showing probity, accountability and being open at all times.
- Ensuring equality, remaining non-judgemental and non-discriminatory.

## Reflection

Candidates initially find the reflection part of the written prioritisation exercise difficult but it is very important and if done correctly it can show you have good insight into your own skills and emotions and can recognise gaps in your knowledge.

Candidates often find that they have left little time for this part of the exercise and therefore we encourage people to have thought about phrases in advance that you may be able to incorporate into your answers. If asked about what you found most difficult you may be able to state you have found some of the tasks did not have enough information to make a good judgement of how to prioritise them. For instance, if you were asked to review a confused patient with no other details given, you could mention that this has an element of ambiguity because it is unclear whether this is acute or chronic confusion and that you would need more details in order to make an informed decision on the urgency of the assessment required.

If asked what you found easy, you could mention that this exercise involved multi-tasking, which is something you have become good at through experience, and therefore you found it easy, especially with the assistance of your colleagues.

## Generic scenarios to prepare for

Each case should be analysed and considered individually on the day. However, to give you ideas on how you may want to prioritise your answers, in **Table 1.2** we suggest approaches to generic scenarios which seem to come up time after time.

There is no right or wrong answer and your own ideas are encouraged. If you feel strongly that something should be done as a first priority, as long as you are able to justify the reason for your choice and it is deemed safe and sensible, you should not lose marks.

It is often easy to decide the first and last priority, but there may be others that seem to have equal importance. It is then down to your own judgement and ability to analyse the problem and explain your choice. If you do change your mind or think you should have done something differently, at the end of the task you should find the opportunity to discuss this in your reflection.

## Top tips

- There are no correct answers but we recommend that you try to put life-threatening clinical issues first.

**Table 1.2 Generic scenarios to prepare for**

| | Clinical scenario | Personal scenario | Family or carer scenario | Healthcare professional scenario | Practical scenario |
|---|---|---|---|---|---|
| **Examples** | Confused patient<br>Unwell patient | Telephone call from your family<br>Application forms<br>Assessment forms<br>Exams | Relative or carer wanting to discuss a patient with you due to complex issues or medical errors | Nurse shouting at a patient<br>GP calling for information<br>Discharge coordinator wanting to discuss a patient | Prescribing<br>Moving your car<br>Sorting out passwords |
| **Suggested priority** | High priority | Medium to low priority | Medium to low priority | Medium priority | Low priority |
| **Notes** | Patient safety to be considered | Depends on nature of scenario; should be placed higher if likely to impact on performance at work | Depends on nature of problem and whether or not patient safety is a concern | Depends on if patient safety is an issue; suggested medium to high priority | If not affecting patient care directly, low priority |

- Use other team members in your answers (where appropriate).
- Appreciate and comment on ambiguity because you will need more detailed information to make decisions in some tasks.
- Aim to make reference to the areas identified in the person specification in your answers.
- Manage your time well.

## Further preparation

You should aim to practise as many exercises as you can under strict exam conditions. Revise your GMC principles and try and incorporate these into your answers.

Think and reflect about things you do every day at work and how you multi-task issues such as dealing with discharge summaries, checking blood test results, prescribing, reviewing patients, talking to relatives, etc. They want you to show that you have real life experience and this will help you produce answers that are realistic, sensible and reflective.

## Reference

General Medical Council. Duties of a doctor. http://www.gmc-uk.org/guidance/good_medical_practice/duties_of_a_doctor.asp, last accessed December 2012.

# Chapter 2

# Written prioritisation: practice cases and model answers

## EXERCISE 1

### Candidate instructions

You are an FY2 doctor in your first month working on a care of the elderly ward. It is now 1600. You must leave by 1700 to go to a seminar where you are presenting your research at 1800 (it takes 1 hour to get to the venue). The various issues below remain outstanding and need to be prioritised for action.

### Your task (30 minutes)

1. To rank each issue in the order in which you intend to deal with it.
2. To justify your decisions and describe what action you will take.
3. To reflect on the challenges posed by this exercise.

All rankings, justifications and comments should be entered and completed within the appropriate boxes on the answer sheet.

You have 30 minutes in total for the exercise. You will be informed when you have 5 minutes left. You should reserve at least 5 minutes to complete the third stage of the task (reflecting on the exercise). This contributes to your assessment and should not be left blank.

### Issues to be ranked

A. The nurse reminds you that there is a confused patient on the ward who has not been assessed.
B. The ward clerk tells you that your mother has called saying she needs to speak to you urgently.
C. The porter phones you to complain that your car is blocking access to the mortuary. He would like you to unblock the access straight away.
D. A GP calls to speak to you as he needs the discharge summary of a patient who was under your care 1 month ago. He has been asked to assess this patient who has become unwell at home.
E. The healthcare assistant reminds you that the family of a patient who was given a drug in error the night before is waiting to speak to you in the family room. The patient had been unwell after this medication error.

## EXERCISE 1 – example answer

1.  **A – The nurse reminds you that there is a confused patient on the ward who has not been assessed.**

    My first priority is to the confused patient. I recognise acute confusion can be an early manifestation of a serious disease requiring urgent care. I would ask the sister to assist me by obtaining observations as I read the history to date. At this point I would also be asking the ward clerk to see if any other team members were available to help with both this patient and the other awaiting tasks. I would discuss this patient with my senior or another colleague, as I am aware I need to leave in 1 hour and this patient may need review or follow up later on. In normal practice, I would utilise all available members of the team to deal with multiple tasks simultaneously. I would also have made sure that my team were aware of my interview well in advance to ensure provisions for adequate ward cover were in place. This is to maximise patient safety without jeopardising my professional development.

2.  **B – The ward clerk tells you that your mother has called saying she needs to speak to you urgently.**

    I would call my mother next. It is very unusual for me to receive personal calls at work and I recognise this could play on my mind and affect my ability and performance. I would need to be aware of this when assessing the confused patient. I would ask the ward clerk to call her back while I was dealing with the first case, to explain that I would be able to call her later but to tell me if it was very urgent. This would at least alleviate my anxieties, allow me to focus on the ill patient and not impact on my limited time. If I needed to leave the hospital because of a family emergency I would tell a colleague immediately and hand over the rest of my jobs. I would also inform my consultant and medical staffing.

3.  **D – A GP calls to speak to you as he needs the discharge summary of a patient who was under your care 1 month ago. He has been asked to assess this patient who has become unwell at home.**

    I would deal with the GP query next, because this task could have a direct impact on a patient's care. This can be done efficiently by asking the ward clerk or pharmacist to fax a copy of the discharge summary urgently to the relevant surgery. I would relay the importance of this issue to whoever does this and would check that this had been completed later on. It is important for the GP to have as much information about the patient as possible, to avoid delaying the patient's medical care and wasting the GP's time. If the discharge summary was easily accessible to me I could also call the GP directly as it may be more efficient and practical to read out the information on the phone. I would also make a note to follow this matter up at a later date to find out the reason for the delay in dispatching the discharge summary, to avoid this happening again in the future.

4.  E – The healthcare assistant reminds you that the family of a patient who was given a drug in error the night before is waiting to speak to you in the family room. The patient had been unwell after this medication error.

This scenario is ambiguous and therefore difficult to prioritise without more information. It is unclear whether the patient needs assessment and still feels unwell; if she is still unwell, she would be a priority. On the other hand, if she is stable and the family require an explanation for the error I would prioritise it last in order to avoid being rushed and interrupted. I would ask the healthcare assistant to obtain this information while I dealt with the confused patient, and also ask the nurse to apologise to the family on my behalf and offer an explanation for my delay. This will ensure that they know I am not ignoring their concerns. In some circumstances, it may be appropriate for a nurse or a pharmacist to talk to the family about the medication error. It is important to deal with such issues quickly to alleviate anxieties and clarify issues honestly. This not only ensures patients and families are treated with respect, but also reduces hospital complaints.

5.  C – The porter phones you to complain that your car is blocking access to the mortuary He would like you to unblock the access straight away.

Blocking the mortuary exit would have huge implications to many people such as staff, funeral directors and bereaved family members. This is an important and urgent issue, but it has been prioritised last because my first duty as a doctor is to patient care. In reality I would ask someone else, possibly a security guard or the porter himself, to move my car for me, making sure he or she was comfortable with this and adequately insured. I would make sure that the car had been moved and, if it had caused any inconvenience, I would personally apologise to the staff it has affected.

## Reflection

1.  **What did you find difficult completing this task and what issues were raised?**

Being asked to formally rank and justify my decisions was very difficult, not only because of the time pressure but also the ambiguity of some of the situations. This task demonstrated how much I trust my colleagues to give important information and reiterated the importance of good communication skills and effective teamwork.

2.  **What did you learn about yourself during this exercise?**

I learned that it is very easy for me to prioritise the tasks where patients are unwell but other non-clinical tasks are much harder. This is probably because they arise less frequently in my everyday practice. In this case, I found it very difficult to prioritise the call from my mother – a situation like this has not yet happened to me and I would expect that if it did it would be a huge distraction. This shows the importance of being flexible and being aware of how your own feelings could affect patient care.

3.  **Would you do anything differently if you were to do this exercise again?**

    If I had to do this task again I may have prioritised the phone call from my mother first, because it is something that I could have done quickly while on my way to assessing the confused patient. I feel this would have meant I would be able to assess this patient more effectively without feeling anxious and distracted.

# EXERCISE 2

## Candidate instructions

You are a surgical FY2 doctor working on a busy hospital ward. It is now 1300. You have booked study leave in order to go on a basic surgical skills course and need to leave by 1400 in order to get there on time. The various issues below remain outstanding and need to be prioritised for action.

## Your task (30 minutes)

1. To rank each issue in the order in which you intend to deal with it.
2. To justify your decisions and describe what action you will take.
3. To reflect on the challenges posed by this exercise.

All rankings, justifications and comments should be entered and completed within the appropriate boxes on the answer sheet.

You have 30 minutes in total for the exercise. You will be informed when you have 5 minutes left. You should reserve at least 5 minutes to complete the third stage of the task (reflecting on the exercise). This contributes to your assessment and should not be left blank.

## Issues to be ranked

A. You are called to review a postoperative patient who has recently undergone an appendicectomy and is complaining of pain.
B. You have an occupational health appointment for hepatitis B and HIV screening, which you were unable to attend at the beginning of your job 1 month ago.
C. A patient who is due to have a laparoscopic cholecystectomy tomorrow needs to have preoperative clerking done.
D. Your hospital password has expired and you need to go to the IT department to reset this in order to access any results, imaging or electronic drug charts.
E. You have agreed to meet your consultant so that he can sign your reference forms for your GP application. He is away on annual leave from tomorrow for 1 month.

# EXERCISE 2 – example answer

1.  **A – You are called to review a postoperative patient who has recently undergone an appendicectomy and is complaining of pain.**

    Assessing this postoperative patient is my first priority. There are many possible causes of postoperative pain in this situation, ranging from peritonitis or wound infection to more benign causes. Whatever the cause of the pain, the patient needs to be assessed promptly and the pain alleviated as soon as possible. I would try to gather a little more information over the telephone and ask the nursing staff to perform observations prior to my arrival. At this point, I would also find out whether any colleagues were available to help me manage this case so that I could move on to the other tasks. For example, the FY1 could initially assess this patient and ask the registrar to review. I am also aware that at this point I have no access to the IT system so I am reliant on another team member to help me review any blood test results and imaging that may be relevant for this patient.

2.  **E – You have agreed to meet your consultant so that he can sign your reference forms for your GP application. He is away on annual leave from tomorrow for 1 month.**

    Once I was confident that the postoperative patient was stable I would try to meet my consultant. Whilst this case does not directly affect patient care it would be quick to do and the thought of failing to get this reference form signed could distract me, which could make me rush the other tasks. If my consultant was not immediately available, I would leave the forms with her secretary, explain the situation and get on with managing the other tasks. If I were able to see my consultant I would also quickly hand over the information about the post-appendectomy patient at the same time.

3.  **D – Your hospital password has expired and you need to go to the IT department to reset this in order to access any results, imaging, or electronic drug charts.**

    It is tempting to leave this task to the end, because I would not want to be delayed in the IT department waiting for my password to be reset while the other tasks remain uncompleted. However, without a password I am unable to review test results and imaging, both of which I will probably need when clerking the preoperative patient. Running around looking for someone to log me in to the computer systems would be a waste of time. Before going to the IT department, I would contact it to see if this could be dealt with over the telephone and, if not, check how long it will take to go there in person. If I were assured that it was a quick task, with no time wasted waiting in a queue, I would go down at this point. If I were informed that it might take 20 minutes I would have to delay this until the following day. I would therefore contact the FY1 and ask him or her to help me clerk the patient.

4.  **C – A patient who is due to have a laparoscopic cholecystectomy tomorrow needs to have preoperative clerking done.**

    This task must be completed this afternoon to ensure that the patient is fit to undergo surgery, has had all the necessary tests done and medications prescribed.

Delay or failure to perform this task could have implications for the patient and colleagues. I need to ensure that this patient is clerked, but this does not necessarily need to be done by me. I have spoken to my FY1 or an FY2 colleague when dealing with the patient in pain, and so at this point I would ask whether they had time to clerk this patient. Before I left I would ensure this had been done.

5. **B – You have an occupational health appointment for hepatitis B and HIV screening, which you were unable to attend at the beginning of your job 1 month ago.**

This task is my last priority. Ensuring screening blood tests are done is extremely important, but from a pragmatic view point it has already been delayed by 1 month and so I do not believe that delaying it for another day would have huge implications. I would contact the occupational health department and let them know that I was struggling to make the appointment and try to reschedule it. I would ensure that I attended the following day and would apologise for wasting their time by cancelling the previous appointment and for not getting these tests done at the start of the job.

## Reflection

1. **What did you find difficult completing this task and what issues were raised?**

I found it hard to prioritise the tasks with such limited information. This demonstrates how important good communication with colleagues is to ensure patient safety and efficient working. Taking the post-appendectomy patient as an example, in normal practice, on receiving this call I would ask the nurse for more information. When was the surgery? What are the observations? How is the patient? From this I would get an idea of the urgency and act appropriately. In the immediate postoperative phase, if the patient was haemodynamically unstable I would immediately inform a senior colleague and rush there myself.

This exercise reinforced the importance of being organised. The afternoon would have been straightforward had I not forgotten to reset my IT passwords, delayed getting my occupational screening done and left the reference signatures to the last minute. Medicine can be unpredictable so it should not be assumed that there will always be time to perform such tasks during working hours without arranging for someone else to cover your work.

2. **What did you learn about yourself during this exercise?**

I learnt that the things that I found challenging and difficult have now changed. One year ago, I would have found dealing with a postoperative patient stressful, but now this seems to be the most straightforward of tasks. I have learned how much I rely on trusting relationships with colleagues, and how important it is to help colleagues out whenever possible so that I feel able to ask for such help myself and delegate things to them.

3. **Would you do anything differently if you were to do this exercise again?**

I think that I would have spent longer working out who was available to help me early on. Once I was confident that the postoperative patient was stable, I could have contacted occupational health to rearrange my appointment, asked the FY1 to clerk the preoperative patient and possibly asked the ward clerk to drop off my reference forms with the consultant's secretary. I could then have gone to IT and returned to the ward to ensure all the tasks had been completed.

# EXERCISE 3

## Candidate instructions

You are an FY2 doctor working on a busy general medical ward. It is now 1600. You must leave by 1700 to collect your child from nursery, which closes at 1730. Your nanny usually does this but she is away on holiday. There is no one else who is available to do this for you.

## Your task (30 minutes)

1. To rank each issue in the order in which you intend to deal with it.
2. To justify your decisions and describe what action you will take.
3. To reflect on the challenges posed by this exercise.

All rankings, justifications and comments should be entered and completed within the appropriate boxes on the answer sheet.

You have 30 minutes in total for the exercise. You will be informed when you have 5 minutes left. You should reserve at least 5 minutes to complete the third stage of the task (reflecting on the exercise). This contributes to your assessment and should not be left blank.

## Issues to be ranked

A. One of your patients has Alzheimer's disease. Her daughter has arrived from abroad to discuss her care.
B. You can hear a healthcare assistant shouting at an elderly patient in the cubicle next to you where you have been taking blood from a patient.
C. The haematology nurse contacts you to inform you that a haematology patient, currently receiving chemotherapy, has developed a fever.
D. The acute medical unit sister tells you that a patient who is being treated for a massive pulmonary embolus is refusing to have his low-molecular-weight heparin injection.
E. You receive a voice message on your mobile from a colleague saying he is running late. This is the second time in the last fortnight in which this has happened, and you need to hand over to him on time today in order to collect your child.

# EXERCISE 3 – example answer

1.  **C – The haematology nurse contacts you to inform you that a haematology patient, currently receiving chemotherapy, has developed a fever.**

    My first priority is to the haematology patient. I recognise that this is could be a life-threatening emergency that needs to be dealt with immediately, especially if the patient is unwell or neutropenic. I would ask the ward clerk to contact my senior registrar while I tend to the patient, as they will need to be involved at an early stage. I would ask the nurse to assist me in order to avoid delays in beginning treatment, such as the administration of antibiotics and fluids. If I was pressured for time and needed to leave, I would ensure the patient is stable, treatment had started and stress the importance of this case when I handed over to a colleague. I would have told my team well in advance that I needed to leave promptly to collect my child, to ensure there was adequate ward cover arranged. This is to make sure I maintain my work life balance and family commitments without compromising patient care.

2.  **E – You receive a voice message on your mobile from a colleague saying he is running late. This is the second time in the last fortnight in which this has happened, and you need to hand over to him on time today in order to collect your child.**

    Having managed the haematology patient I would deal with this issue, because there are implications on patient care if there is no medical cover available when the doctor is late. I would initially find out how delayed my colleague is, explain that I will be unable to stay late to cover (normally I would be willing to work flexibly to help colleagues and ensure adequate cover). If he cannot make it on time, I would contact medical staffing (if none of my other team members were able to cover). I would also want to address the reasons for the repeated delays and find out if my colleague needed additional support. This needs to be dealt with in a timely and sensitive manner. Given that this is such a time-pressured situation I would leave this until the following day.

3.  **D – The acute medical unit sister tells you that a patient, who is being treated for a massive pulmonary embolus, is refusing to have his low-molecular-weight heparin injection.**

    With this limited information, it is difficult to accurately prioritise this task. It is unclear whether the patient is stable; if he is not, this needs to be prioritised higher. There is also no information about how long the patient has been in hospital and whether treatment started prior to this. If the patient were stable I would need to have an open discussion with the patient regarding the refusal of treatment, exploring his ideas and concerns and highlighting the potential consequences of failure to achieve optimal anticoagulation. This task could be delegated to a senior nurse, medical colleague or pharmacist in the first instance.

4.  **B – You can hear a healthcare assistant shouting at an elderly patient in the cubicle next to you where you have been taking blood from a patient.**

    The healthcare assistant shouting at the patient is an important issue to deal with.

Patients should receive the highest quality of care and should be treated with respect at all times. This is particularly important in vulnerable groups who rely wholly on the care of others. I would ask the ward sister to take responsibility for dealing with this to ensure it does not happen again. Although this behaviour is inexcusable, it is important to keep an open mind and try and educate the assistant about how to behave towards patients and explore why they were shouting and whether they need support.

5.  **A – One of your patients has Alzheimer's disease. Her daughter has arrived from abroad to discuss her care.**

I would leave this task until last to ensure I had adequate time to discuss important issues about this patient's future care with her daughter. I would ensure the nursing staff informed her of the reason for my delay. If she did not want to wait I could arrange another mutually convenient time to speak to her, either face-to-face or by telephone. When speaking to patients or their relatives it is important to have read the notes and be up-to-date with the situation. It may be possible for another member of my team to deal with this. I would therefore ask the nurse or ward clerk to see if anyone else was available while I dealt with the first case.

## Reflection

1.  **What did you find difficult completing this task and what issues were raised?**

I found this exercise very difficult, not only because of the time pressure, but also the ambiguity of some of the situations. It was certainly easy to prioritise acute clinical cases first, as this is something I do on a daily basis in my clinical practice. It was much harder to prioritise those where immediate patient safety was not at risk. Some of the issues raised related to professionalism at work (i.e. the colleague being late for a shift). I have little experience with this sort of situation and I need more experience in dealing with potentially underperforming colleagues or those who may be having difficulty.

2.  **What did you learn about yourself during this exercise?**

This task showed me how much I trust my colleagues to give important information and demonstrated the importance of good communication skills and strong teamwork. I learned how much more difficult it is to deal with these situations without knowing which of my colleagues were available to help. This task reinforced how important it is to not to try to deal with everything yourself.

3.  **Would you do anything differently if you were to do this exercise again?**

If I were to repeat this task I would try to obtain more information about each case and establish who was available to help earlier. In this way I would be able to delegate some tasks and ensure that they were all dealt with efficiently and carefully, without rushing.

# EXERCISE 4

## Candidate instructions

You are an FY2 doctor working on a busy geriatric ward. It is now 1600. You must leave in 1 hour to attend a talk you have agreed to give at the medical school you attended. The talk is on the application process for final year medical students. The various issues below remain outstanding and need to be prioritised for action.

## Your task (30 minutes)

1. To rank each issue in the order in which you intend to deal with it.
2. To justify your decisions and describe what action you will take.
3. To reflect on the challenges posed by this exercise.

All rankings, justifications and comments should be entered and completed within the appropriate boxes on the answer sheet.

You have 30 minutes in total for the exercise. You will be informed when you have 5 minutes left. You should reserve at least 5 minutes to complete the third stage of the task (reflecting on the exercise). This contributes to your assessment and should not be left blank.

## Issues to be ranked

A. Your registrar has asked you to meet him to go through some case-based discussions. This meeting has been planned since last week. Your deadline for completion of this exercise is imminent.
B. You are called by the mortuary to complete a cremation form for a patient who died 2 days ago.
C. You are called by the nursing staff to review an elderly patient on the ward who is refusing her afternoon medications.
D. Your crash bleep goes off stating there is a cardiac arrest in the acute assessment unit.
E. The physiotherapist has asked you to attend the multidisciplinary team discharge planning meeting for the patient who has been refusing medications.

## EXERCISE 4 – example answer

1.  **D – Your crash bleep goes off stating there is a cardiac arrest in the acute assessment unit.**

    I would immediately respond to the arrest bleep. If I were the first doctor to arrive I would assess the patient using an ABC (airway, breathing, circulation) approach and if this were a true arrest situation, commence cardiopulmonary resuscitation. I would ask the nurses to get the crash trolley (if it were not already there) and delegate tasks, such as getting intravenous access and managing the patient's airway, to the appropriate people. There are usually many arrest call responders and it may be possible to leave the arrest early in order to continue with the other tasks. I would discuss this with my registrar and FY1, who also carry the arrest bleep, at this opportunity. I would explain the time-pressured situation and see if some of the other tasks could be delegated or deferred.

2.  **C – You are called by the nursing staff to review an elderly patient on the ward who is refusing her afternoon medications.**

    This case is difficult to prioritise because of the lack of information but, on balance, I feel it needs to be dealt with urgently. The patient may be on critical medications; furthermore, her refusal to take the medications could represent an acute confusion. I would try to get more information from the nursing staff when I received this call to help me triage these tasks more effectively. At the arrest call I would ask the ward FY1 or an FY2 colleague to review this patient, but if this were not possible I would ask one of the nurses to talk to the patient to get more information prior to my arrival.

3.  **B – You are called by the mortuary to complete a cremation form for a patient who died 2 days ago.**

    It is important to deal with this task as soon as possible. Delays in the completion of this form may have consequences on the deceased patient's family and delay plans to transfer the body to the undertakers. It is usual practice for the doctor who signed the death certificate to complete the cremation form, so if I had not completed this I would ask the mortuary to see if the appropriate doctor was available. When I received this call I would ask how urgently the form was needed. Often there is no rush and it would be a better use of my time to deal with this the following day. If I caused any delay in getting this done I would apologise to the mortuary staff and explain the reasons why.

4.  **E – The physiotherapist has asked you to attend the multidisciplinary team discharge planning meeting for the patient who has been refusing medications.**

    It is very important that a member of the medical team attends this valuable meeting to ensure the safe discharge of this patient. Unfortunately the other tasks would take priority and I would liaise with my colleagues to ensure that someone else from the medical team could attend. It is important that the patient is assessed prior to this meeting so up-to-date information is available for making the discharge decision (especially as this patient is refusing to take her medications). Failure for any medical team member to attend could delay discharge. If no one else is available to attend this meeting I would go myself, apologise for any delay and ask whether it would be possible to give my input early and leave before the meeting was completed.

5.  **A – Your registrar has bleeped you to ask you to meet him to go through some case-based discussions. This meeting has been planned since last week. Your deadline for completion of this exercise is imminent.**

    Workplace-based assessments are extremely important for my ongoing professional development but given the time-pressured situation, this is my last priority on this occasion. It can take 30 minutes to discuss a single case and this should be done at an appropriate time when we would not be disturbed. I would ask my registrar whether we could defer this meeting when we met at the arrest call. I would make sure that this meeting was conducted at a time when there would be adequate cover on the ward and I would not be rushing off to give a talk to medical students.

## Reflection

1.  **What did you find difficult completing this task and what issues were raised?**

    Being asked to rank these tasks and justify my decisions was difficult. I was extremely pressured for time (replicating the scenario) and the cases were ambiguous. This showed how much I rely on good communication between colleagues to ensure that tasks are triaged effectively. I found it particularly hard to prioritise the task involving the patient refusing medications. There is such a range of reasons why this may be and I ended up having to act according to a worse-case scenario policy.

    This exercise demonstrated that it is impossible to deal with everything myself and it is extremely important to recognise and utilise the skills of other team members to allow tasks to be completed simultaneously.

2.  **What did you learn about yourself during this exercise?**

    This exercise highlighted that I feel most comfortable dealing with medical problems because I have had experience doing this since starting work as a doctor. I found it difficult to think of workable solutions to the remainder of the problems and think I have a tendency to try to do too much myself – not wanting to burden my colleagues. In fact, the best patient care is achieved if team members work closely together and share work according to abilities.

3.  **Would you do anything differently if you were to do this exercise again?**

    On reflection I think I would have tried to get to, or arranged for a colleague to attend the discharge meeting before I completed the cremation form. It is unlikely that a delay in filling in the cremation form would impact greatly on the family's plans, as most cremations take place at least 1 week after death. However, a failure to attend, or lateness attending, the discharge meeting would impact more on the patient and colleagues. This also has wider implications for the trust.

# EXERCISE 5

## Candidate instructions

You are an oncology F2 doctor working on a busy hospital ward. It is now 1200. You must leave by 1300 to go to your brother's graduation. The various issues below remain outstanding and need to be prioritised for action.

## Your task (30 minutes)

1.  To rank each issue in the order in which you intend to deal with it.
2.  To justify your decisions and describe what action you will take.
3.  To reflect on the challenges posed by this exercise.

All rankings, justifications and comments should be entered and completed within the appropriate boxes on the answer sheet.

You have 30 minutes in total for the exercise. You will be informed when you have 5 minutes left. You should reserve at least 5 minutes to complete the third stage of the task (reflecting on the exercise). This contributes to your assessment and should not be left blank.

## Issues to be ranked

A.  The husband of a patient who has just been diagnosed with inoperable gastric cancer has asked to speak with you about his wife.
B.  You have been asked to meet the palliative care nurse on the ward. She has agreed to do a practical tutorial on setting up a syringe driver. This is one of the competencies you need to demonstrate during your job.
C.  You are asked by the day assessment unit sister to review a patient with known lung cancer, who has come in feeling very short of breath.
D.  A physiotherapist, who you saw crying earlier that day, has asked you to meet with her so she can speak to you in confidence.
E.  You have been asked by a medical student on your firm if you could teach him how to take blood samples.

## EXERCISE 5 – example answer

1.  **C – You are asked by the day assessment unit sister to review a patient with known lung cancer, who has come in feeling very short of breath.**

    I would prioritise this potentially life-threatening situation first. This patient requires urgent assessment and treatment. I would do the initial review and request the necessary investigations. At this point I would also ask the ward clerk to find out which other colleagues were available to help me with both this and the other tasks. If the patient was very unwell I would call the critical outreach team (depending on what services are available) to update them about the patient and ask for regular review. I would also inform my registrar of this admission, to ensure that the patient was reviewed once I had finished my shift.

2.  **A – The husband of a patient who has just been diagnosed with inoperable gastric cancer has asked to speak with you about his wife.**

    This is another extremely important and sensitive issue. When dealing with such situations it is important not only to care for the patient, but also to give as much support as possible to the family. This is devastating news, and may be unexpected, therefore this is an issue that deserves uninterrupted time so that the family feel free to open up and ask questions.

    One possibility would be to contact my registrar or consultant to ask if they would be able to speak to the patient and her husband. If this were not possible, I would ask the sister in charge to speak to them and let them know that I would be coming shortly. They would then know that their request has not been ignored and would give them time to think about what they would like to ask. By this point I would hopefully have been in touch with my colleagues and would ask one of them to hold my bleep so that I was not disturbed.

3.  **D – A physiotherapist who you saw crying earlier that day has asked you to meet her so she can speak to you in confidence.**

    I would try to meet the physiotherapist next. I do not think it is appropriate to delegate this task to anyone else as she has specifically asked to speak to me. I would spend time exploring why she was upset but, as I am aware that I have to leave shortly, I would make sure that I arranged a time to meet her the next day to discuss things further. This would hopefully make her feel that she is not alone and that people are there to help her. It is important to show compassion for our colleagues, as the work place can be a very difficult and stressful place at times.

4.  **B – You have been asked to meet your palliative care nurse on the ward who has agreed to do a practical tutorial on setting up a syringe driver. This is one of the competencies you need to demonstrate during your job.**

    This is a very important issue. Setting up a syringe driver can be tricky and I would want to ensure I could do this before my next on-call shift. It is also very kind of the nurse to take time out of her day to teach me. It would probably be more appropriate to rearrange this for a time when I was less rushed and I would try to speak to the nurse when I was on the ward dealing with the breathless patient, to see if we could find another mutually convenient time.

5.  **E – You have been asked by a medical student on your firm if you could teach him how to take blood samples.**

    Medical students can sometimes feel a bit lost and ignored so it is important to make them feel like they are a part of the team. I would explain that I am a busy today and need to go to my brother's graduation, but give him the bleep number of my house officer to see if he is free to teach him. If not, then he can shadow my house officer and learn how to do other jobs, and also re-review the patient who has come in short of breath. I would also suggest spending some time with a phlebotomist. I would apologise, but hopefully the alternative would also be a valuable learning experience and I would offer to teach him on an alterative, less time-pressured, day.

## Reflection

1.  **What did you find difficult completing this task and what issues were raised?**

    I found it difficult to prioritise these tasks, as they were all important for different reasons. Patient safety must always come first, but the other tasks were much more complex. Several issues were raised, such as education for me and for students, breaking bad news and caring for colleagues. All are issues that need addressing and prioritising them into a sensible order was very challenging.

2.  **What did you learn about yourself during this exercise?**

    I learned how important it is to be aware of who is available on your team. The scenario is rather ambiguous, in that it has not told you who you have on your team, or what day it is – it could be a Saturday.

    I also learned that when you have to leave at a specific time, you need to tell everyone in your team well in advance. Tasks can then be split and bleeps handed over in good time. That way, if emergencies come to light the appropriate cover has already been arranged.

3.  **Would you do anything differently if you were to do this exercise again?**

    Once I had ensured that the breathless patient was stable. I would spend a few moments establishing who was available to help before planning how best to utilise my available colleagues. That way we can tackle all of the tasks more efficiently. I would also have liked to approach the physiotherapist immediately when I saw her crying, to offer support at that point rather than leaving it until later.

# EXERCISE 6

## Candidate instructions

You are an FY2 doctor working on the acute assessment unit. It is now 1500. You must leave by 1600 to go to a physiotherapy appointment as you are currently recovering from a fractured ankle. Your consultant is aware of this and you obtained permission from medical staffing and your team in advance. Missing this appointment is not an option, nor is arriving late. The various issues below remain outstanding and need to be prioritised for action.

## Your task (30 minutes)

1. To rank each issue in the order in which you intend to deal with it.
2. To justify your decisions and describe what action you will take.
3. To reflect on the challenges posed by this exercise.

All rankings, justifications and comments should be entered and completed within the appropriate boxes on the answer sheet.

You have 30 minutes in total for the exercise. You will be informed when you have 5 minutes left. You should reserve at least 5 minutes to complete the third stage of the task (reflecting on the exercise). This contributes to your assessment and should not be left blank.

## Issues to be ranked

A. You are called to the ward to write up a patient's regular medications. The patient was admitted to the ward the previous day and has not yet had his antihypertensive medication.
B. The ward sister bleeps you to ask you to review a patient who has started fitting on the ward. The patient is known to have epilepsy.
C. You have been asked to call the care of the elderly consultant on another ward about a patient you saw the day before.
D. A patient you discharged yesterday following an acute exacerbation of chronic obstructive pulmonary disease has called the ward wanting to speak to you about his medications.
E. The coffee shop calls you to let you know that you left your wallet there this morning.

## EXERCISE 6 – example answer

1.  **B – The ward sister bleeps you to ask you to review a patient who has started fitting on the ward. The patient is known to have epilepsy.**

    I would attend to this patient immediately. Urgent administration of medication may be needed if the fit fails to stop spontaneously. The patient is also at risk of sustaining injuries during the fit and it is important to establish why it has occurred. The patient is known to suffer from epilepsy but I would want to ensure that his antiepileptic medications have been prescribed and given correctly, and that there was no reason why the seizure threshold has reduced (i.e. due to an infection or from new medications). On arrival I would ask a nurse to assist me while I make an initial assessment and instigate treatment. If the seizure continued, senior help would be needed so I would ask a nurse to contact my registrar and the ITU team.

2.  **A – You are called to the ward to write up a patient's regular medications. The patient was admitted to the ward the previous day and has not yet had his antihypertensive medication.**

    This needs to be dealt with fairly urgently. The patient probably has missed a day of medications and may have unstable hypertension as a result. I would ask the nurse what the blood pressure and pulse are, to ensure there is no imminent risk. If the blood pressure was not dangerously high I would ask my house officer to write the appropriate medications onto the drug chart and ensure that a dose was given this afternoon. At a later point, when I had more time, I would ensure I looked into why the medications had not been written up correctly on admission.

3.  **C – You have been asked to call the care of the elderly consultant on another ward about a patient you saw the day before.**

    As I am already by the phone, I would then call the care of the elderly consultant. I would want to do this as quickly as possible to ensure that any questions the consultant had were answered as soon as possible, and also because I know that I would worry about the nature of the call. Wondering whether I had done something wrong, or missed a diagnosis would play on my mind. Consultants do not often call, so this must be something important and should not be ignored.

4.  **D – A patient you discharged yesterday following an acute exacerbation of chronic obstructive pulmonary disease has called the ward wanting to speak to you about his medications.**

    There are many different reasons why the patient has called. Perhaps he does not understand the new treatment plan, something may have been prescribed erroneously or he may be feeling unwell again. I would ask the senior sister if she would kindly speak to the patient to find out more information while I dealt with the other tasks. I would prioritise this higher if the patient seemed unwell. If the patient wanted to ask a question about medication, the ward pharmacist may be best placed to answer any queries. The pharmacist also has access to discharge summaries, and so has the information available and is often able to give detailed answers. If, however, there are still queries I would speak to the patient myself once I had completed the above tasks.

5. **E – The coffee shop calls you to let you know you left your wallet there this morning.**

   On receiving this call I would thank the staff for informing me and ask them to keep it safe until I could collect it. I could easily pop into the coffee shop on the way out of the hospital as long as it was still open at 4 pm. If not, I would ask the coffee shop staff whether they would mind dropping it off at the hospital reception. Clearly it is important to get my wallet back but I should not need it over the next hour and so this would be my last priority.

## Reflection

1. **What did you find difficult completing this task and what issues were raised?**

   I found it difficult to prioritise these tasks with limited information available. I ended up having to make assumptions that I usually would not in clinical practice. I also found it difficult to order the tasks when, in reality, I would try to tackle them simultaneously.

   Several issues were raised in this task. It demonstrated how important good communication is between team members, and also how important it is to have trusting working relationships with colleagues. I felt awkward when writing my justifications because I felt that I was continuously asking colleagues to do things for me. I realise that this would be easier in everyday practice, when I know my team members would be aware that my reason for delegating is because I am extremely busy rather than lazy.

2. **What did you learn about yourself during this exercise?**

   I learned that no matter how hard you try to be organised, medicine is extremely unpredictable. The best way to tackle this is to arrange a handover time with your team well in advance. In this way, if emergencies do crop up 20 minutes before you need to leave, someone else is available to deal with it.

   I also learned that it is hard to balance personal situations and work priorities, such as in the case with the lost wallet. Sometimes these situations have to be prioritised highly because worry or stress may affect work performance.

3. **Would you do anything differently if you were to do this exercise again?**

   On reflection I would probably deal with the call to the patient first. A nurse or pharmacist could make the initial call and I would arrange for this while on my way to review the fitting patient. I think that the call from the consultant could be delayed because the patient is on the ward, under medical care and I would hope that the consultant would have expressed suitable urgency if the patient were at immediate risk. I would also try to involve other team members earlier so that all of the tasks could be completed without rushing to leave at 4 pm.

# EXERCISE 7

## Candidate instructions

You are a junior doctor working on a busy general surgical ward. It is now 1600. You must leave by 1700 as you are going on holiday and are catching a flight to Prague that evening. You must leave promptly in order to get to the airport in time. The various issues below remain outstanding and need to be prioritised for action.

## Your task (30 minutes)

1. To rank each issue in the order in which you intend to deal with it.
2. To justify your decisions and describe what action you will take.
3. To reflect on the challenges posed by this exercise.

All rankings, justifications and comments should be entered and completed within the appropriate boxes on the answer sheet.

You have 30 minutes in total for the exercise. You will be informed when you have 5 minutes left. You should reserve at least 5 minutes to complete the third stage of the task (reflecting on the exercise). This contributes to your assessment and should not be left blank.

## Issues to be ranked

A. You are asked by the nursing staff to write up a patient's warfarin dose for the day. The international normalised ratio (INR) is available for this.
B. You are called to review a patient on the ward who has started to complain of chest pain. The patient was supposed to go home this morning but was apprehensive about leaving the hospital.
C. You hear an FY1 doctor on the ward shouting at a patient who is refusing to allow blood samples to be taken.
D. You are called by your consultant, who is currently in clinic, to bring down the notes that he has left on the ward for a patient he is about to review. He says it is urgent.
E. A GP has called to speak to you to discuss a discharge summary you wrote about one of his elderly patients who has a complex medical history.

# EXERCISE 7 – example answer

1.  **B – You are called to review a patient on the ward who has started to complain of chest pain. The patient was supposed to go home this morning but was apprehensive about leaving the hospital.**

    I would attend to this patient first. There are many causes of chest pain, some of which are life-threatening and/or time-sensitive, and so reviewing this patient is my first priority. On receiving this call I would ask the nurse for additional information. Nurses are well trained to recognise a sick patient and I would want to briefly establish how the patient is and ask the nurse to perform observations and an ECG. I would then review the patient, take a history, perform an examination and review the ECG. The patient may still be safe to go home (for example, if this was a muscular pain) but my response would clearly depend on my interpretation of the cause of the pain. If I had any concerns I would inform my registrar, the ward sister (as the bed may no longer be available) and I would also inform the on-call team to ensure that the patient was reviewed and appropriate investigations (for example, a troponin test) were carried out.

2.  **C – You hear an FY1 doctor on the ward shouting at a patient who is refusing to allow blood samples to be taken.**

    It is very important to deal with this as soon as possible. It is not appropriate to show frustration or anger towards a patient and I would want to understand why this had happened. I would ask to speak to the FY1 privately, explain what I had overheard and try to understand why it had happened. The FY1 may be struggling with his workload, be overly stressed or feel unsupported. Due to time pressures, I may have to agree to meet him the following day to discuss how to deal with these situations but I think it is important for someone to speak to the patient this evening and make sure that he has not been affected by the incident. The ward sister may be able to do this, or could give me some background information on the incident.

3.  **D – You are called by your consultant, who is in clinic, to bring down the notes that he has left on the ward for a patient he is about to review. He says it is urgent.**

    This needs to be dealt with urgently to avoid wasting the consultant or the patient's time. It is also important for patient safety because it is would be difficult for the consultant to make a thorough assessment without the notes. Given all of the other tasks that I need to tackle, this would be the best one to delegate – possibly to the ward clerk or porter. I would explain to the consultant that I will ensure that the notes are brought to the clinic urgently and I would follow this up to make sure that there are no problems. This task can be completed quickly and simultaneously alongside other tasks and so I would try to sort this out immediately upon receiving the consultant's call.

4.  **E – A GP has called to speak to you to discuss a discharge summary you wrote about one of his elderly patients who has a complex medical history.**

    My next priority would be to call the GP back. This task perhaps requires a little more time than the preceding two tasks, because the GP may need more details about the patient's admission. It needs to be dealt with this afternoon while the GP practice is still open and I would apologise for any delay returning the call. If I felt anyone else knew the patient, for example the FY1, I would ask this person to call the GP and see if all of the GP's concerns could be answered. I would then ensure that the FY1 had been able to deal with this and find out what information was needed. If any information was unclear or had been omitted from the discharge summary I would learn from this.

5.  **A – You are asked by the nursing staff to write up a patient's warfarin dose for the day. The international normalised ratio (INR) is available for this.**

    This would be my last priority. The patient certainly needs the correct warfarin dose, but as warfarin tends to be given in the evening there would be no benefit in doing this sooner. On receiving this call I would ask the nurse whether on this occasion he could contact the FY1 or another SHO to do this. The following day I would ensure that the warfarin was prescribed for the next few days (as long as daily INR checks were not required).

## Reflection

1.  **What did you find difficult completing this task and what issues were raised?**

    The information given in the tasks was ambiguous, making it difficult to effectively prioritise. This highlights the importance of good communication, with appropriate information passed between colleagues to enable fast and accurate triaging of the tasks.

    Several issues were raised. There is only 1 hour to get a lot of jobs done, but missing my flight is not an option for me as I believe in maintaining a good work life balance. Another issue of respecting patients was highlighted. I heard an FY1 shouting at someone, but do not know the whole story. In reality, if I heard someone shouting at a patient, I would intervene immediately to diffuse the situation.

2.  **What did you learn about yourself during this exercise?**

    I learned how important it is to be aware of your team and what services are available to you. I have this knowledge of the hospital where I am currently based, as I have been there for the past few years. This task demonstrated the challenges I am likely to face when starting in a new unit or hospital, as each one is different. There are always people around to help, such as phlebotomists, pharmacists, critical outreach members, senior colleagues, etc. It is important to recognise that there is always support available.

    I also learned how important it is to be organised. In this scenario, making sure my team knew that I needed to leave at a certain time and arranging the handover is imperative. This would ensure that I could leave on time, and that patient safety is not jeopardised in order to do this.

3.  **Would you do anything differently if you were to do this exercise again?**

    On reflection, I would try to deal with more things concurrently. While I was on my way to the ward to see the patient with chest pain, I could probably ask the senior sister on the ward to deal with the FY1 who is shouting (chances are she probably heard it herself and is already on her way to deal with it), and also quickly ask the ward clerk to take the notes down to my consultant. This way, three tasks can be accomplished relatively quickly. I would then attend to the patient with chest pain, and after assessment, ask my colleague or the SHO to meet up to handover the case, ensuring continuity of care for my patient.

# EXERCISE 8

## Candidate instructions

You are a junior doctor working on a busy hospital ward. It is now 1600. You must leave by 1700 to catch a train to Edinburgh where you are being interviewed for a job the following day. The various issues below remain outstanding and need to be prioritised for action.

## Your task (30 minutes)

1. To rank each issue in the order in which you intend to deal with it.
2. To justify your decisions and describe what action you will take.
3. To reflect on the challenges posed by this exercise.

All rankings, justifications and comments should be entered and completed within the appropriate boxes on the answer sheet.

You have 30 minutes in total for the exercise. You will be informed when you have 5 minutes left. You should reserve at least 5 minutes to complete the third stage of the task (reflecting on the exercise). This contributes to your assessment and should not be left blank.

## Issues to be ranked

A.  You saw your registrar in the doctor's mess kissing another registrar the night before, whilst on call. She is married with children and was very embarrassed. She has asked you to meet her to discuss what happened.
B.  You need to write a fitness to work note for a patient who was admitted with pneumonia and is now ready for discharge.
C.  You are asked to review a patient on the ward who is threatening to jump out of a window. He is shouting on the ward repeatedly saying he wants to die.
D.  You realise that you have left your ID badge and mobile phone in the canteen.
E.  You are called by the switchboard operator, who asks you to call your mother, who has left a message for you because she could not get through to you on your mobile.

## EXERCISE 8 – example answer

1. **C – You are asked to review a patient on the ward who is threatening to jump out of a window. He is shouting on the ward repeatedly saying he wants to die.**

   I would deal with this immediately. I would ask the nurse to also contact my registrar and hospital security, as the patient seems to be at significant risk. If the patient has a known mental health condition I would also ask the nurse to contact the psychiatric duty manager urgently. Upon arriving on the ward I would make an immediate appraisal of the situation. Is the patient approachable? Is the window open? Is there immediate danger? I would then try to talk to the patient to understand what has been going on – I would try to find out whether this is an acute delirium or a presentation of a psychiatric condition and manage it accordingly. Sectioning under the mental health act may be necessary if the patient tries to leave the ward and the psychiatric team are likely to need to be involved.

2. **A – You realise that you have left your ID badge and mobile phone in the canteen.**

   I would try to collect my ID and mobile phone from the canteen next. This would not take a great deal of time and without ID, moving around the hospital becomes very difficult. I do not think it would be realistic to expect anyone else to get these for me, especially given the situation unfolding on the ward, and so this would have to be delayed until the suicidal patient was stable. I also know that my mother has been trying to call me and she has probably left a message that may indicate the urgency of the call. Receiving this message may save me from having to call back immediately.

3. **E – You are called by the switchboard operator, who asks you to call your mother, who has left a message for you because she could not get through to you on your mobile.**

   Unless my mother had left a message on my phone I would be very worried about the nature of her call. She has never contacted me via the switchboard before and I therefore suspect she needs to speak to me urgently. Delaying calling her would play on my mind and so prevent me from attending to the other tasks with a clear head. Again, I couldn't really delegate this task to anyone else but I would quickly establish the nature of the call and then hopefully I would be able to move on to the final two tasks without significant delay.

4. **B – You need to write a fitness to work note for a patient who was admitted with pneumonia and is now ready for discharge.**

   This task needs dealt with quickly in order to avoid delaying the discharge and blocking the bed. If the patient leaves without this note it would also put an unnecessary burden on the patient's GP. The FY1 could do this task and I could ask the ward clerk to bleep her and convey this message. If she had any concerns or questions about how long the note should be for we could discuss this over the phone. By delegating this task it could be completed much earlier and free up time for me to address the other tasks.

5.  **A – You saw your registrar in the doctor's mess kissing another registrar the night before, whilst on call. She is married with children and was very embarrassed. She has asked you to meet her to discuss what happened.**

    I would deal with this issue as my last priority because it does not have anything to do with clinical care and the other tasks seem more urgent. Ideally, I would try not to arrange a meeting of this sort on a day when I know I have to leave and I am busy. I would call my registrar, explain the situation to her and ask if she was free to help me with some of the awaiting tasks, such as the suicidal patient. I would try and reschedule the meeting with her and apologise for this, as I am aware she is embarrassed and worried about what happened. It is important to keep good relations with colleagues and I am generally not a judgemental person. I would try my best to relay this to my registrar in order to be able to continue working well with her as part of a team.

## Reflection

1.  **What did you find difficult completing this task and what issues were raised?**

    I found it very difficult to prioritise my mother's call. This does not usually happen to me and I know that if this were a real situation I would be extremely worried. This is especially true as she tried to call the switchboard. This highlighted the importance of looking after my own wellbeing at work, and I realised how something like this could indirectly impact on patient care if I was not completely focussed, which is why I prioritised it highly.

2.  **What did you learn about yourself during this exercise?**

    I also learnt that it is important to use other members of your team when you do have multiple tasks to complete in a short space of time; delegation is an important aspect of working as part of a team and trying to do too much on your own can cause unnecessary delays and maybe even more work in the long-term.

    I also realised that I have very little experience of patients who are suicidal in the acute setting and I would probably have felt a bit lost when I reviewed the patient. I would not know what to do with regards to physical constraint or sedation if this was required. This has highlighted an area of weakness in my knowledge that I need to address.

3.  **Would you do anything differently if you were to do this exercise again?**

    If I had to complete this exercise again, I would call my registrar earlier to explain that I could not meet her, and I would ask her to come and review the suicidal patient. I know she is free because we had agreed to meet; her help with some of the tasks would be very much appreciated. I could have called my mother through the switchboard, if the operator was happy for me to do so, to find out if my mother's call was serious and then I could have dealt with my ID and phone as a lower priority.

# EXERCISE 9

## Candidate instructions

You are a urology FY2. It is now 1600. You must leave by 1700 to go to take your mother to a hospital appointment. You must leave promptly to be there on time. The various issues below remain outstanding and need to be prioritised for action.

## Your task (30 minutes)

1. To rank each issue in the order in which you intend to deal with it.
2. To justify your decisions and describe what action you will take.
3. To reflect on the challenges posed by this exercise.

All rankings, justifications and comments should be entered and completed within the appropriate boxes on the answer sheet.

You have 30 minutes in total for the exercise. You will be informed when you have 5 minutes left. You should reserve at least 5 minutes to complete the third stage of the task (reflecting on the exercise). This contributes to your assessment and should not be left blank.

## Issues to be ranked

A. You are called by a social worker who has some concerns about an elderly housebound woman who was discharged home yesterday by your team.
B. You are called by your FY1 who is struggling to insert a urinary catheter into a patient on the ward.
C. You are called by medical staffing as you have not handed in your hours monitoring form that was due in this morning.
D. You are asked to review a patient on the ward who had a radical prostatectomy 2 days ago. He has started shouting and has become confused and agitated.
E. Your registrar has asked to meet you to discuss an audit you had agreed to do with her.

## EXERCISE 9 – example answer

1. **D – You are asked to review a patient on the ward who had a radical prostatectomy 2 days ago. He has started shouting and has become confused and agitated.**

   Dealing with this patient is my first priority. This presentation may indicate a surgical complication such as sepsis or may be a sign of something unrelated, for example alcohol withdrawal. In addition to the immediate risk to the patient, his agitation may be distressing for the other patients on the ward. On being asked to come and review the patient I would ensure that the nursing staff had the notes ready and if possible (without putting their safety at risk) ask them to obtain observations. If the patient presented a risk to staff or patients I would ask the nurse in charge to contact security. I would attend to the patient as quickly as possible to try and ascertain the cause of his delirium and manage this accordingly. If possible I would ask another member of my team, possibly my registrar, to help me.

2. **B – You are called by your FY1 who is struggling to insert a urinary catheter into a patient on the ward.**

   I would deal with this task next. Although the catheter may not need to be inserted urgently the failed attempts are likely to have been distressing for the patient and it would be best to complete this as soon as possible. It would also provide an excellent teaching opportunity for the FY1. I would advise the FY1 that I would be attending once I had dealt with the agitated patient – this would be important so that the patient was not left waiting uninformed mid-procedure. I would also ask the FY1 to see if the registrar was available to help complete this task sooner.

3. **A – You are called by a social worker who has some concerns about an elderly housebound woman, who was discharged home the day before by your team.**

   I would deal with this as soon as possible. While I was dealing with the tasks above I would ask the ward clerk to contact the social worker to explain that I am currently busy but would call back. The ward clerk may be able to find out the concerns and the urgency of the question. The social worker may also indicate that one of the ward nurses or the FY1 would be able to help, and the ward clerk would be able to forward this call on to the appropriate person.

4. **E – Your registrar has asked to meet you to discuss an audit you had agreed to do with her.**

   This task is prioritised fourth because it does not immediately affect patient care. Audit is an essential part of clinical governance that ensures high quality of care. I know how hard it is to find time to meet colleagues to discuss audits and research and so I would not want to lose this opportunity. I would call my registrar whilst dealing with the agitated patient and explain the situation. She may be able to help and by working together to complete the tasks we would probably have enough time to hold a brief meeting.

5.  **C – You are called by medical staffing as you have not handed in your hours monitoring form that was due in this morning.**

    This is my last priority. Patient care is not immediately affected and a delay in handing in the completed monitoring form, whilst frustrating, should not affect the results or outcome. When called I would explain that I was extremely busy on the ward and ask if a faxed copy would be acceptable. If the answer was 'no', I would have to apologise and explain that I could hand in the form either that evening, on my way home, or the following morning, unless there was somebody available to collect it from the ward.

## Reflection

1.  **What did you find difficult completing this task and what issues were raised?**

    It is difficult to safely prioritise tasks with such limited information. Assumptions have to be made which, in clinical practice, I would not normally make. Whenever I am bleeped or called I always obtain further information to help understand the urgency of the task; without this direct colleague-to-colleague communication, prioritising becomes very difficult. I also found it hard delegating without knowing the team I am working in. Ordering the tasks was challenging – usually I would deal with a medical emergency and then spend a few minutes gathering information, delegating the remaining less urgent tasks and dealing with some of them simultaneously, rather than moving from one to another in this manner.

2.  **What did you learn about yourself during this exercise?**

    I realised while doing this task that I am systematic in my approach to clinical work. I recognise that my priority is always to put patient safety first and I recognise my limitations and ask for help early when I am struggling to cope with the workload.

3.  **Would you do anything differently if you were to do this exercise again?**

    With the luxury of more information relating to the tasks at hand, I would have been able to make better judgements on what needed to be done. I could have argued that the clinical cases could have been dealt with later on while I very quickly made a few phone calls, but this again would depend on having more information about the safety of the patient who was confused and more details about the circumstances of the patient needing a catheter – for instance, is there painful urinary retention? If there were enough team members around, I could have spent a few minutes delegating tasks. This would have resulted in more efficient use of everyone's time rather than leaving a registrar waiting for me to have a meeting that is unlikely to occur given the short space of time I had.

# EXERCISE 10

## Candidate instructions

You are a medical FY2 working on a busy acute hospital ward. It is now 1500. You must leave by 1600 to go to a play in which your partner is acting in. The various issues below remain outstanding and need to be prioritised for action.

## Your task (30 minutes)

1. To rank each issue in the order in which you intend to deal with it.
2. To justify your decisions and describe what action you will take.
3. To reflect on the challenges posed by this exercise.

All rankings, justifications and comments should be entered and completed within the appropriate boxes on the answer sheet.

You have 30 minutes in total for the exercise. You will be informed when you have 5 minutes left. You should reserve at least 5 minutes to complete the third stage of the task (reflecting on the exercise). This contributes to your assessment and should not be left blank.

## Issues to be ranked

A. You are asked to speak to the relatives of a patient who had a subarachnoid haemorrhage and is currently on ventilatory support in the ITU.
B. You are called to the emergency department to review a patient who fell off a ladder, sustaining a head injury. His Glasgow coma score is fluctuating between 10 and 14.
C. Your registrar has asked you to meet him on the ward to carry out a lumbar puncture under his supervision so you can get a directly observed procedural skills (DOPS) assessment done.
D. The nurses on the ward ask you to do a discharge summary for a patient who was told she could go home this morning. She has been waiting for 4 hours and is very angry.
E. You need to go to radiology to arrange an urgent CT pulmonary angiogram (CTPA) for an inpatient who has become short of breath, and who has a $PO_2$ of 9 kPa on a blood gas test.

## EXERCISE 10 – example answer

1. **B – You are called to the emergency department to review a patient who fell off a ladder, sustaining a head injury. His Glasgow coma score is fluctuating between 10 and 14.**

   My first priority is assessing this patient with a reduced Glasgow coma score. This suggests he has a serious, potentially life-threatening condition and there is a risk that his airway could become compromised. I would ask the ward staff to contact my registrar, as this patient should not be managed alone, and ask the nurses do basic observations and blood tests. This patient needs to be stabilised and a brain CT should be performed. The patient may have an intracranial bleed and may continue to deteriorate. If I confirmed a low Glasgow coma score I would also involve the intensive treatment unit team as he may need intubation.

2. **E – You need to go to radiology to arrange an urgent CT pulmonary angiogram (CTPA) for an inpatient who has become short of breath, and who has a $PO_2$ of 9 kPa on a blood gas test.**

   I would deal with this task next, as it is important that a diagnosis is made promptly to ensure the patient receives optimal treatment. This may include anticoagulation for a pulmonary embolism. I would ensure the patient was being assessed and managed appropriately by someone on my team; then I would find out if my FY1 was available to request this investigation, ensuring that the FY1 had all the information required by the radiologist. This could be more time-efficient than going to radiology myself, although if I needed an urgent brain CT for the patient with a reduced Glasgow coma score I could request both of these together. If no one was available to help I could also call the radiologist from the ward to discuss the case and arrange the CTPA, rather than going to the department in person.

3. **C – Your registrar has asked you to meet him on the ward to carry out a lumbar puncture under his supervision so you can get a directly observed procedural skills (DOPS) assessment done.**

   Opportunities for training such as this are infrequent. Whilst I could explain to the registrar that I am busy and ask him to go ahead and do it himself, this may impact on future patient care when I am still unable to do this procedure competently. I would therefore prioritise this highly. I would have already involved my registrar in the care of the patient with the reduced Glasgow coma score and so, if we were both busy, the lumbar puncture might have to be delayed. If the procedure was urgent, then I would ask a competent colleague if he or she was able to do it and I would make an effort to find similar training opportunities in the future.

4. **D – The nurses on the ward ask you to do a discharge summary for a patient who was told she could go home this morning. She has been waiting for 4 hours and is very angry.**

   Although I recognise that discharge delays such as this are extremely frustrating, this can only be prioritised fourth due to the urgent nature of the other tasks. I would ask the nurses to apologise to the patient and explain the situation. I would also ask them to bleep the house officer and see if he is available to do the discharge summary faster than I could.

5.  **A – You are asked to speak to the relatives of a patient who had a subarachnoid haemorrhage and is currently on ventilatory support in the ITU.**

    I have prioritised this task last for various reasons. This task does not involve patient care directly but it is very important that relatives of patients who are very unwell are spoken to in a sensitive and timely fashion, with efforts made to minimise any chance of interruption. It is for this reason that I would want the other tasks completed before sitting down with the relatives, so I can hand my bleep to someone else. I would ask the ITU nurse to explain to the relatives that I will be delayed and ensure that they are comfortable in the family room while they wait for me. I could also ask the nurses if a more senior member of the team, ideally the consultant, was free to deal with this. It is sometimes more appropriate for senior colleagues to have these sorts of discussions about critically unwell patients as they are the most experienced and likely to be able to answer potentially difficult questions about issues surrounding prognosis.

## Reflection

1.  **What did you find difficult completing this task and what issues were raised?**

    I found this task difficult because I deemed many of the jobs to be clinically important and urgent. In reality I would spend 5 minutes delegating tasks if a situation like this were to arise, for example getting my FY1 or another FY2 to help with ordering tests while I saw the patient with the fluctuating Glasgow coma score. This exercise demonstrated that it is almost impossible to do all of these things on your own and that without knowing who else is around, it is difficult to decide how best to proceed. It highlights the importance of good teamwork. It is also difficult to make decisions about certain tasks unless you are fully informed about what is going on. For example, it is not clear whether or not the hypoxic patient is being dealt with on the ward or not. It would be inappropriate to leave the patient, who may be unstable, to go to radiology.

2.  **What did you learn about yourself during this exercise?**

    I realised that I am systematic in my approach to clinical work. I recognise that my main duties are as a doctor where my priority is always to put patient safety first. I recognise my limitations and ask for help early when I am struggling to cope with the workload. I also learned that my strong relationships with colleagues are vitally important to good teamwork.

3.  **Would you do anything differently if you were to do this exercise again?**

    If I could do this again I probably would have dealt with the family of the patient in ITU first. I would not have dealt with it by myself but at least I would have called to explain that I would not be able to come immediately and therefore ask that they try to find someone else to speak to them so that they are not kept waiting.

# EXERCISE 11

## Candidate instructions

You are a medical FY2 on the general and endocrinology ward. It is now 1600 on Friday afternoon. You must leave by 1700 to catch a flight to go to Scotland where you are attending a wedding that weekend. Being late is not an option. The various issues below remain outstanding and need to be prioritised for action.

## Your task (30 minutes)

1. To rank each issue in the order in which you intend to deal with it.
2. To justify your decisions and describe what action you will take.
3. To reflect on the challenges posed by this exercise.

All rankings, justifications and comments should be entered and completed within the appropriate boxes on the answer sheet.

You have 30 minutes in total for the exercise. You will be informed when you have 5 minutes left. You should reserve at least 5 minutes to complete the third stage of the task (reflecting on the exercise). This contributes to your assessment and should not be left blank.

## Issues to be ranked

A. You are asked to meet your consultant to discuss a complaint letter that has been received. You have been named in the complaint letter and have to write a response within 14 days.
B. You are asked to do the 2-hourly blood tests for a patient who is currently undergoing an oral glucose tolerance test.
C. You are called by the ward sister who tells you that an insulin-dependent diabetic patient is drowsy and has a blood glucose of 1.6 mmol/L.
D. A patient's daughter has asked to speak to you. She is upset about her mother's care and is shouting at a healthcare assistant who is trying to clean the patient.
E. You need to go to security to have the battery of your bleep replaced as it has stopped working.

# EXERCISE 11 – example answer

1. **C – You are called by the ward sister to tell you that an insulin-dependent diabetic patient is drowsy and has a blood glucose of 1.6 mmol/L.**

   I would first review this hypoglycaemic patient as this is a medical emergency and must be dealt with immediately. On receiving this call I would ask the sister to administer fast-acting dextrose gel to the patient, stop any insulin infusion (if running) and perform observations. Once the patient had been stabilised it would be important to assess how this hypoglycaemia had occurred and address any causative factors. I would also consider asking the diabetic specialist nurses to assess this patient, ensure that regular blood sugars are being taken and ask for the team to be called if any hypoglycaemic episodes occur again. I would also make a point of handing over to the evening staff to ensure this patient is reviewed.

2. **E – You need to replace the battery of your bleep at security as it has stopped working.**

   Being easily contactable while at work is important for patient safety. Without a functioning bleep I could be unaware of sick patients whilst the ward staff wondered why I had not answered their calls. I would therefore deal with this urgently. Ideally I would not leave the ward myself. I could either ask the ward clerk whether there is a supply of batteries or whether it is possible to get the battery changed for me while I dealt with the next tasks.

3. **B – You are asked to do the 2-hourly blood tests for a patient who is currently undergoing an oral glucose tolerance test.**

   These blood tests need to be taken within set time intervals. If these intervals are missed the test results cannot be interpreted and the test would need to be repeated. A competent colleague could do these blood tests and so I would see if a trained nurse, medical student or phlebotomist was free to do this. If no one else was available, I could ask the nursing staff if they were able to prepare the equipment I needed before I got there to allow me to take the sample quickly and efficiently.

4. **D – A patient's daughter has asked to speak to you. She is upset about her mother's care and is shouting at a healthcare assistant who was trying to clean the patient.**

   I would want to deal with this issue as soon as possible as this patient's daughter is clearly distressed and her shouting on the ward could adversely affect the patient, staff and other patients on the ward. I would ask the ward sister to take the patient's daughter into the relative's room, explain my delay and see if she could find out more information about the nature of the complaint. If another member of my team was available I would ask him or her to deal with this to reduce the delay but if not I would ensure that I went as soon as possible. Dealing with complaints correctly at this stage can reduce family anguish, address the family's concerns and reduce the chance of a formal complaint being made.

5.  **A – You are asked to meet your consultant to discuss a complaint letter that has come through from a patient. You have been named in the complaint letter and have to write a response within 14 days.**

    I would have wanted to deal with this urgently but I felt that the other cases took priority. I would ask the ward clerk to explain that I had a lot of things to deal with and would be there as soon as possible. There is no immediate rush to write a response but this complaint would play on my mind and I would certainly want to discuss it before going home. It can also take time to write a measured response and to get an opinion from a defence union if needed.

## Reflection

1.  **What did you find difficult completing this task and what issues were raised?**

    I found it difficult to prioritise speaking to the consultant about the complaint letter. I am aware that there are often few opportunities to meet and I would not want to spend days wondering what the complaint was about. I would also be mindful that the anxiety this sort of situation creates may affect my ability to deal with the other tasks effectively, and I would have prioritised this higher if this seemed to be occurring.

2.  **What did you learn about yourself during this exercise?**

    I am generally very comfortable dealing with medical emergencies such as hypoglycaemia, but I find dealing with angry patients or relatives more challenging, This is probably because these are skills developed through experience and it is often left to more senior members of the team to deal with complaints when they arise. I think I possibly have a tendency to get a little defensive when dealing with angry patients or complaints when in fact it is important to listen to the complaint, try to understand what has happened and learn from it. I shall try to bring this into my clinical practice and gain more experience during my training.

3.  **Would you do anything differently if you were to do this exercise again?**

    I would have tried to deal with a few things simultaneously earlier on. Whilst I was dealing with the hypoglycaemic patient, I could have contacted the switchboard with the information that my bleep was not functioning and asked for my calls to be diverted. I could also have asked the ward sister to see if someone else was available to obtain blood samples from the patient undergoing a glucose tolerance test rather than trying to find someone myself.

# EXERCISE 12

## Candidate instructions

You are a paediatric FY2 working on a busy hospital ward. It is now 1300. You did the late shift last night and are due to finish today at 1400. You have booked yourself on a basic paediatric life support course at a nearby hospital that afternoon and need to leave promptly to make it on time. The various issues below remain outstanding and need to be prioritised for action.

## Your task (30 minutes)

1. To rank each issue in the order in which you intend to deal with it.
2. To justify your decisions and describe what action you will take.
3. To reflect on the challenges posed by this exercise.

All rankings, justifications and comments should be entered and completed within the appropriate boxes on the answer sheet.

You have 30 minutes in total for the exercise. You will be informed when you have 5 minutes left. You should reserve at least 5 minutes to complete the third stage of the task (reflecting on the exercise). This contributes to your assessment and should not be left blank.

## Issues to be ranked

A. You are asked to attend a meeting organised by the registrar in charge of your rota. He is hoping to rearrange the rota and needs to know everyone's availability.
B. You are asked to review a child admitted with a viral-induced wheeze. He is not feeding well and has become more tachypnoeic.
C. You need to complete your online application form for GP specialty training as the deadline closes in the next hour.
D. You are asked to write up intravenous fluids for a 7-week-old baby who is awaiting surgery for pyloric stenosis.
E. You are called by the pharmacist to discuss a medication error on a discharge summary you completed this morning.

# EXERCISE 12 – example answer

1. **B – You are asked to review a child admitted with a viral-induced wheeze. He is not feeding well and has become more tachypnoeic.**

   I would review this patient first because worsening tachypnoea is a concerning sign and this patient may need urgent treatment. Children can deteriorate rapidly and so I would ask the ward clerk to contact my registrar and inform her of the situation. I would also ask a nurse to review the child with me to help obtain observations. I know that I would not want to leave this patient until he was stable; thus, if I was delayed with this task, I would ask a competent colleague to assess and prescribe fluids for the preoperative baby. Once stable the child will require regular reviews. I would ask the nurses to perform regular observations and to inform me, or my colleague once I had handed over, if there was any further deterioration.

2. **D – You are asked to write up intravenous fluids for a 7-week-old baby who is awaiting surgery for pyloric stenosis.**

   I recognise that it is crucially important that this patient receives appropriate hydration prior to surgery. As I mentioned above, I would see if a colleague was available to do this; if not I would review the notes, check when the baby's last blood gas had been taken and clinically assess the hydration status. To help me do this I would check whether the baby had been weighed recently and if not I would ask one of the paediatric nurses to do this. I would then prescribe fluids but I would also inform my paediatric surgical and anaesthetic colleagues, as correct fluid balance in babies is crucial.

3. **C – You need to complete your online application form for GP specialty training as the deadline closes within the next hour.**

   After dealing with the two ill patients I would address this task. I think I would struggle to concentrate on the other remaining tasks unless this was completed, as the implications of not submitting it are enormous. Clearly this is not a task that can be done by anyone else, but I would hope that it would be a quick task which could easily be completed and allow me to finish the outstanding jobs. I would immediately assess how long it was likely to take and if it seemed that it would take longer I would contact both the pharmacist and registrar to see if the remaining tasks could be delayed or delegated to another colleague.

4. **E – You are called by the pharmacist to discuss a medication error on a discharge summary you completed this morning.**

   Upon receiving this call I would ask the pharmacist whether this was something that needed to be dealt with immediately. The fact that the pharmacist had picked up on an error seems to suggest that the patient is not at risk, but this error would certainly be something I would want to look into and learn from. I would make every effort to deal with this by 2 pm but if this was impossible I would ask one of my colleagues to contact the pharmacist to see if they could help. The following day I would contact the pharmacist myself.

5.  **A – You are asked to attend a meeting organised by the registrar in charge of your rota. He is hoping to rearrange the rota and needs to know everyone's availability.**

    I have opted to deal with this problem last because, although a delay in completing the rota would be frustrating to all involved, it would not immediately impact on patient care. I know that writing rotas can be very hard and extremely time consuming and so would apologise to my registrar and explain the situation. I would also ask whether I could give my colleague a note with my availabilities to take to the meeting. It is probably not essential that I attend and this would allow the meeting to progress and the rota to be organised.

## Reflection

1.  **What did you find difficult completing this task and what issues were raised?**

    It is extremely difficult prioritising these tasks with such little information about the cases or staff that are available to assist me. I know that this would be a very stressful hour and recognised that the thought of failing to submit my GP application would play on my mind, so I opted to complete this fairly early. I think this certainly showed that medicine is unpredictable and it is not wise to leave non-clinical tasks with deadlines to the last minute or to arrange courses that start immediately after work.

2.  **What did you learn about yourself during this exercise?**

    The first thing that this task highlighted was my lack of postgraduate paediatric experience. This is something I would hope to address during my GP training. This task also showed how much I rely on colleagues to work effectively together. The information given is very brief and usually I would gather more information to help me prioritise effectively.

3.  **Would you do anything differently if you were to do this exercise again?**

    I would spend time getting more information earlier on to allow me to prioritise more effectively. Once the two ill patients were stabilised I would contact the registrar in charge of the rota and the pharmacist and explain the time-pressured situation. I hope this would alleviate some of this pressure and allow me to complete my GP training application in slightly less stressful circumstances.

# EXERCISE 13

## Candidate instructions

You are a junior doctor working on an acute medical ward. It is now 1600. You must leave by 1700 to play in a hockey match. Missing this is not an option. The various issues below remain outstanding and need to be prioritised for action.

## Your task (30 minutes)

1.  To rank each issue in the order in which you intend to deal with it.
2.  To justify your decisions and describe what action you will take.
3.  To reflect on the challenges posed by this exercise.

All rankings, justifications and comments should be entered and completed within the appropriate boxes on the answer sheet.

You have 30 minutes in total for the exercise. You will be informed when you have 5 minutes left. You should reserve at least 5 minutes to complete the third stage of the task (reflecting on the exercise). This contributes to your assessment and should not be left blank.

## Issues to be ranked

A   You are asked to speak to a medical student, admitted yesterday after falling off his bike, about the fact that he mentioned to you that he had taken drugs. You included this in his clerking notes. He now claims he was joking at the time he said it.

B.  A patient on the ward, who is a GP himself, has asked to speak to you about the nutritional status of the opposite him patient on the ward.

C.  A patient informs the senior nurse on the ward that her medications are written incorrectly on her drug chart. Her GP has faxed her medications list and it does not correspond with her drug chart. You have been asked to verify this and amend it as appropriate.

D.  A healthcare assistant has asked to speak to you about her boyfriend, who is also a healthcare assistant on the ward. She has told you it is about the fact that he used to look at child pornography.

E.  You are asked to review a patient who has started passing blood per rectum. She has just been started on clopidogrel after having a non-ST elevation myocardial infarction (NSTEMI) 3 days ago.

## EXERCISE 13 – example answer

1. **E – You are asked to review a patient who has started passing blood per rectum. She has just been started on clopidogrel after having a non-ST elevation myocardial infarction (NSTEMI) 3 days ago.**

   I would deal with this patient as my first priority as she is having a potentially life-threatening gastrointestinal bleed. She is at high risk of serious bleeding because of the anticoagulation treatment with clopidogrel. In addition, any significant blood loss may cause further damage to her myocardium. When informed about this patient I would ask the nurses for further information because I would want to know the volume of blood loss and her cardiovascular observations. If a significant bleed had occurred, I would inform my senior colleague at this point in case the patient needed to have an emergency endoscopy. I would ask another colleague (my house officer or senior nurse) to help and I would site a large-bore cannula and send blood samples for FBC, clotting and cross-match. If the patient was stable I would request that a colleague review her regularly while I managed the other tasks; I would also inform the cardiologists of the potential need to stop the anticoagulation treatment.

2. **C – A patient informs the senior nurse on the ward that her medications are written incorrectly on her drug chart. Her GP has faxed her medications list and it does not correspond with her drug chart. You have been asked to verify this and amend it as appropriate.**

   I would deal with this issue next because the patient may come to harm if she receives the wrong medications. I would try to get additional information over the telephone. What has been written incorrectly? What medications have been missed? Clearly my response would then be changed by the information. If, for example, an emollient was missed off, or a sleeping tablet not prescribed I could delay dealing with this (or ask a colleague to deal with it – possibly my house officer). If an important drug had been given incorrectly or at the incorrect dose, however, a more urgent response would be necessary. On arriving on the ward I would review the notes, the drug chart and the information sent by the patient's GP. I would work out whether the patient had been put at risk and would act accordingly. To do this I may need to speak to a pharmacist. I would then inform the patient and explain what actions had been taken to resolve the mistake, and I would ask the ward sister to fill out an incident form so that lessons could be learned from this.

3. **A – You are asked to speak to a medical student, admitted yesterday after falling off his bike, about the fact that he mentioned to you that he had taken drugs. You included this in his clerking notes. He now claims he was joking at the time he said it.**

   I would talk to the medical student next as he may be very distressed and worried about the consequences of my clerking. I suspect that he has decided to say he was joking about taking drugs because he is worried about the impact of this admission from the previous night, but it is important to keep an open mind and try to get the full story. In advance of speaking to the medical student I would want to clarify the rules regarding this situation – to do this I could contact the advice line provided by my medical defence union. I do not think it is possible to delete an entry in the notes unless it is an entry added in error. The only option may be to add an additional entry detailing the clarification. Of course I would want to spend time talking to him, assure him that our consultation was confidential and try to establish if he had taken drugs. If he had, he may need support and advice; the fact that he is a medical student should not mean he feels unable to seek professional help for fears of jeopardising his career. As a medical student, drug-taking is unlikely to have put patients at risk however there are clear probity issues.

4.  **B – A patient on the ward, who is a GP himself, has asked to speak to you about the nutritional status of the patient opposite him on the ward.**

    I would deal with this situation next. It is very important to hear the concerns of another professional in this situation but I did not prioritise this higher because it does not seem as though the patient is at immediate risk. I would explain to the ward sister that I was extremely busy but would come to see him. The ward sister may even be able to deal with the situation without the need for a doctor to become involved. I would ensure that the nurse was aware that to disclose any medical information about the patient would be breaching confidentiality.

5.  **D – A healthcare assistant has asked to speak to you about her boyfriend, who is also a healthcare assistant on the ward. She has told you it is about the fact that he used to look at child pornography.**

    This issue is a very serious criminal allegation and certainly needs to be dealt with but I have prioritised it last because I feel it will take time, it should not be rushed and I do not think patients are at immediate risk. I would deal with this issue myself because I can appreciate that it must have been very hard for the healthcare assistant to tell me this sensitive information and so it would be wrong to ask someone else to deal with it without her consent.

    I am aware that I do not have a great deal of experience dealing with issues like this but would try to listen and explore exactly what had happened in the past. I would certainly need to get senior help to investigate this allegation and ideally the healthcare assistant should, if she felt comfortable with this, speak directly to a line manager so the information was passed on 'first-hand'. If I really did not have time to deal with this issue I could also apologise to the healthcare assistant and arrange a meeting before work the following day.

## Reflection

1.  **What did you find difficult completing this task and what issues were raised?**

    Prioritising these tasks with very little information and therefore significant ambiguity was very hard. It showed how important good communication between colleagues is. This would certainly have been a very difficult and stressful afternoon. I found dealing with the non-clinical issues particularly tricky. With both issues A and D, I struggled to think of the correct course of action and so certainly felt it would be inappropriate to delegate to a more junior team member. I think the main thing that this task showed me was how important teamwork is, and that without it none of these tasks could be managed efficiently. It also showed me that it is impossible to deal with everything thrown at me and it may be necessary to delay dealing with some tasks in order to handle them thoroughly.

2.  **What did you learn about yourself during this exercise?**

    I realised that although I feel competent at a clinical level there are gaps in my knowledge in certain non-clinical areas. I do not know how I would answer questions about whistleblowing polices and procedures, where I would find out such information and who, in the hospital setting, I would speak to. This task certainly highlighted this learning need and also the importance of seeking help when dealing with new, unfamiliar clinical or managerial issues.

3.  **Would you do anything differently if you were to do this exercise again?**

    I do not feel I would change the order of my priorities. I may, however, have taken slightly different actions to complete some, for example postponing the meeting with the healthcare assistant while I spoke with my defence union and possibly doing the same with the medical student. I could have called for help from my team a little earlier in the exercise to try and get some tasks dealt with concurrently to optimise efficiency. For example, I could have asked the pharmacist to deal with the medications while I was dealing with the bleeding patient.

# EXERCISE 14

## Candidate instructions

You are a junior doctor working on a busy hospital ward. It is now 1200. You must leave by 1300 to attend a revision course that you have previously booked study leave for. The various issues below remain outstanding and need to be prioritised for action.

## Your task (30 minutes)

1. To rank each issue in the order in which you intend to deal with it.
2. To justify your decisions and describe what action you will take.
3. To reflect on the challenges posed by this exercise.

All rankings, justifications and comments should be entered and completed within the appropriate boxes on the answer sheet.

You have 30 minutes in total for the exercise. You will be informed when you have 5 minutes left. You should reserve at least 5 minutes to complete the third stage of the task (reflecting on the exercise). This contributes to your assessment and should not be left blank.

## Issues to be ranked

A. Your consultant bleeps you to remind you that you are meeting him to fill out your online assessment forms for your end of placement review.
B. A nurse calls you to tell you that a patient has fallen on the ward and needs to be assessed. The fall was not witnessed.
C. You are called by your house officer who asks you to speak to the family of a patient who died unexpectedly the night before following a myocardial infarction.
D. A nurse on the acute admissions ward calls you to tell you a patient would like to self-discharge. He was admitted the night before with an asthma attack and has said that he was told he could go home. This is not documented in the notes and his 'to take outs' (TTOs) have not been done.
E. The ward clerk tells you that medical staffing have left a message. Your bank details are incorrect and they are unable to process your pay. Today is the deadline and they need you to come and sign some forms. If you cannot do this today your pay will not go into your account this month.

## EXERCISE 14 – example answer

1. **B – A nurse calls you to tell you that a patient has fallen on the ward and needs to be assessed. The fall was not witnessed.**

   A patient who has fallen may have sustained significant injuries and may also have an underlying condition that lead to the fall. This case is difficult and shows how much one relies on the additional information our colleagues give us to prioritise effectively. With the limited information provided here my first priority is to this patient. I would ask the nursing staff to obtain observations and perform an initial assessment of this patient. I would also ask the nurse on the admissions ward to tell the patient planning to self-discharge to wait until I could see him. I could then assess the patient, take a concise history of the incident and make sure no injures had occurred before moving on to the other tasks.

2. **D – A nurse on the acute admissions ward calls you to tell you a patient would like to self-discharge. He was admitted the night before with an asthma attack and has said he was told he could go home. This is not documented in the notes and the 'to take outs' (TTOs) have not been done.**

   This patient clearly had a significant asthma exacerbation. While he may feel better, he could quickly relapse. It is important to assess him properly and, if he is found to be well enough to go home, ensure that he has the correct medications and is instructed to seek help if any deterioration occurs (safety netting). Initially, it may be possible for my house officer to see this patient and organise the TTOs so that the patient could be reassured that if fit for discharge, there would be minimal delay. This is important as it has wider financial implications for the trust and also affects nurses and pharmacists, who may need to prepare the take home medications.

3. **C – You are called by your house officer, who asks you to speak to the family of a patient who died unexpectedly the night before following a myocardial infarction.**

   This is obviously a very distressing time for the family and I would be keen to not keep them waiting. When the house officer called I would ask him to see if my consultant or registrar was available to see the family. This would free up time for me to complete the other tasks and it is also good practice for the most senior available member of the team to speak to family members in these circumstances. If nobody else could do this, I would ask the ward sister to inform the relatives that I was on my way, apologise for my delay, and give them an approximate time of my arrival. I would read the notes carefully and hand my bleep to a colleague prior to meeting them to minimise any interruption.

4. **A – Your consultant bleeps you to remind you that you are meeting him to fill out your online assessment forms for your end of placement review.**

   When bleeped by my consultant I would explain that I had urgent jobs to do and see if it were possible to reschedule this meeting. I recognise that I have a responsibility to keep up-to-date with my assessments but this should not be done when rushed.

Rescheduling would also allow me to spend more time on the other tasks. In addition, I could also use this as an opportunity to see if my consultant was available to speak to the grieving relatives. If the consultant were unable to reschedule I would prioritise this fourth and hope that by involving other team members to help me complete the tasks I would have time to attend this review.

5.  E – The ward clerk tells you that medical staffing have left you a message. Your bank details are incorrect and they are unable to process your pay. Today is the deadline and they need you to come and sign some forms. If you cannot do this today your pay will not go into your account this month.

    Whilst it may be frustrating to be paid late, the other cases take priority in this situation. I would quickly ask the ward clerk to phone medical staffing with my correct bank details; if this was not possible I would approach them the next day and hope that they were willing to organise a cheque for the first month's pay.

## Reflection

1.  **What did you find difficult completing this task and what issues were raised?**

    Being asked to formally rank and justify my decisions was very difficult, not only because of the time pressure but also the ambiguity of some of the situations. This exercise showed how important it is to have adequate cover on the wards to ensure patient safety is not put at risk. It has also highlighted the importance of strong teamwork.

2.  **What did you learn about yourself during this exercise?**

    This task demonstrated how much I trust my colleagues to give important information and demonstrated once again the importance of good communication skills and strong teamwork. By delegating tasks appropriately it is possible to achieve a great deal in limited amount of time. It is also important to appreciate my own limitations – in this case I felt that it would be better for a senior colleague to talk to the recently bereaved relatives and I made it a priority to facilitate this.

3.  **Would you do anything differently if you were to do this exercise again?**

    I think that I engaged different colleagues effectively in this task but if I were to repeat it I would spend a minute before attending to any case obtaining more information, so I could prioritise the tasks most effectively. I may also have asked medical staffing to meet me with the forms on the ward, if they were willing to do this, to quickly sign the forms.

# EXERCISE 15

## Candidate instructions

You are an FY2 on a busy hospital ward and have to leave in 1 hour to catch a flight to go to Northern Ireland where you are presenting a poster. The various issues below remain outstanding and need to be prioritised for action.

## Your task (30 minutes)

1.  To rank each issue in the order in which you intend to deal with it.
2.  To justify your decisions and describe what action you will take.
3.  To reflect on the challenges posed by this exercise.

All rankings, justifications and comments should be entered and completed within the appropriate boxes on the answer sheet.

You have 30 minutes in total for the exercise. You will be informed when you have 5 minutes left. You should reserve at least 5 minutes to complete the third stage of the task (reflecting on the exercise). This contributes to your assessment and should not be left blank.

## Issues to be ranked

A.  A medical student tells you that a patient with chronic obstructive pulmonary disease (COPD) is having difficulty breathing and may need more oxygen.
B.  A woman is at the nurses' station crying, saying she can't cope with her daughter at home if her daughter is discharged from hospital today.
C.  A 16-year-old girl, who came in with a paracetamol overdose last night, has locked herself in the toilet with a knife.
D.  Your FY1 Dr Jay is heard shouting at a patient behind curtains whilst the patient's son is next to you waiting to complain about his mother's care.
E.  The ward sister wants to talk to you about Dr Jay offering cocaine to a nurse last night during the on-call shift.

# EXERCISE 15 – example answer

1.  **C – A 16-year-old girl, who came in with a paracetamol overdose last night, has locked herself in the toilet with a knife.**

    I would deal with this patient first as patient safety is at risk and she could be in imminent danger. I would ask the nursing staff to call my senior colleague, the on-call psychiatry team, and security as a matter of urgency, in case the toilet door needs to be forcefully opened. I would also ask them to inform the surgical team of this case pre-emptively. Once I am satisfied that enough senior support had arrived I would move on to deal with the other urgent jobs.

2.  **A – A medical student tells you that a patient with chronic obstructive pulmonary disease (COPD) is having difficulty breathing and may need more oxygen.**

    As soon as I was confident that the suicidal girl is being dealt with and is safe, I would review the patient with COPD. When the medical student told me that the patient needed more oxygen I would have asked him to bleep another member of the team who could assess this patient while I was dealing with the suicidal girl. The team member would also be able to carry out further investigations, including a blood gas test, if needed. This issue needs to be prioritised highly because it is not simply a case of increasing the patient's oxygen. The cause of the respiratory distress should be established and oxygen needs to be used with care in most patients with COPD.

3.  **D – Your FY1 Dr Jay is heard shouting at a patient behind curtains whilst the patient's son is next to you waiting to complain about his mother's care.**

    This is an issue that needs to be dealt with promptly. Patients should receive the highest quality of care and must be treated with respect at all times. In reality, if I heard a colleague shouting at a patient I would probably intervene immediately, apologise to the patient and ask to speak to Dr Jay in private at a later point. In this situation (where there are two sick patients to deal with first) I would ask the ward sister to intervene and then I would make it a priority to speak to Dr Jay and the patient or patient's relative once the other tasks had been dealt with.

4.  **B – A woman is at the nurses' station crying saying she can't cope with her daughter at home if her daughter is discharged from hospital today.**

    Whilst it is important to deal with this situation as soon as possible the patient is not at immediate risk on the ward and so I have prioritised this fourth. Her mother is clearly upset and should be showed compassion. It would be appropriate for a senior nurse to take the mother aside and try to establish what problems are happening at home and why she feels unable to cope. I would make it clear that the patient should not be discharged until all the facts had been established and the appropriate services informed. Once I had dealt with the three tasks above I would then try to meet the nurse and find out what the problems were before meeting the mother herself.

5. **E – The ward sister wants to talk to you about Dr Jay offering cocaine to a nurse last night during the on-call shift.**

   This is a very difficult and sensitive matter. There is an allegation that a doctor has potentially been using the illegal drug cocaine, offering it to other staff, and this doctor has also been heard shouting at a patient. The first task is to ensure that Dr Jay stops working immediately to minimise clinical risk. On receiving this call I would ask the sister whether she feels able to discuss this with a more senior staff member. This would allow me to focus on the other tasks but would also be more appropriate given the seriousness of the allegation. I would then ensure that Dr Jay's work was covered for the remainder of the day by seeing if any other FY1s were available to take his bleep and also by informing my registrar.

## Reflection

1. **What did you find difficult completing this task and what issues were raised?**

   I found the ambiguity of some of these cases difficult. The lack of information made it hard to prioritise them safely and I was forced to make judgements that in everyday practice I would not make. I have not dealt with an underperforming colleague before and this made it difficult for me to imagine how I would manage this situation. Whilst I recognised that patient safety could have been at risk and that he needed to stop working immediately, I was unsure who would be best placed to take this matter further.

2. **What did you learn about yourself during this exercise?**

   I have learnt that I still have gaps in my knowledge regarding certain clinical areas such as psychiatry. The task involving the suicidal girl demonstrated this. I realise that it is important to evaluate and reflect on areas of weakness in order to gain broad experience during GP training. This exercise also showed how much I rely on teamwork and good communication in my clinical practice.

3. **Would you do anything differently if you were to do this exercise again?**

   I found it difficult to carry out this task due to the time pressures. If given the opportunity to do this again I would prioritise things in the same order but I would also have asked the nurse to immediately inform the consultant about Dr Jay as this is a difficult issue requiring immediate senior input.

# Chapter 3

# Consultation skills: introduction

## Introduction

The selection centre requires you to complete three 10-minute consultations:

1. A consultation with a patient.
2. A consultation with a patient's relative.
3. A consultation with a non-medical colleague.

These will be situations that you should be able to deal with as a doctor with at least 18 months of postgraduate experience. They will not involve any physical examination, and clinical expertise is not being specifically assessed (this has already been tested in your written examinations). Each case is examined in isolation from the others: the examiners will usually mark the same case throughout the morning or afternoon session.

The three consultation exercises are designed to see how you interact with patients and what skills you have developed in your training so far. Consulting effectively is fundamental for general practitioners and so, whilst undergraduate and hospital medicine largely focuses upon diagnosis and treatment, general practice training emphasises the need to communicate and consult effectively with patients.

Your ability to engage the patient and actively adjust your behaviour and language according to the needs of the consultation is being assessed. To help you do this effectively, and to help you score highly, this chapter discusses a few key areas to focus on. It does not pretend to be a consultation skills manual; indeed, GP training applicants are not expected to fully understand the mechanics of a consultation. The three simulated consultations require a different approach to the basic history, examination and investigation template often taught at undergraduate level, an approach tailored to the real circumstances of clinical practice.

Consider the selection centre process in detail and focus your preparation directly toward the assessment. The old adage 'practice makes perfect' is never more relevant than here and is why we have included so many cases in this revision guide.

## The set-up

Deaneries use many types of venues: you may be performing the consultations in a hotel room or a small seminar room in a conference centre, for example.

You will be invited into a room where the examiner will usually already be present. You will have a few moments to rearrange the chairs (**Figure 3.1**), to facilitate

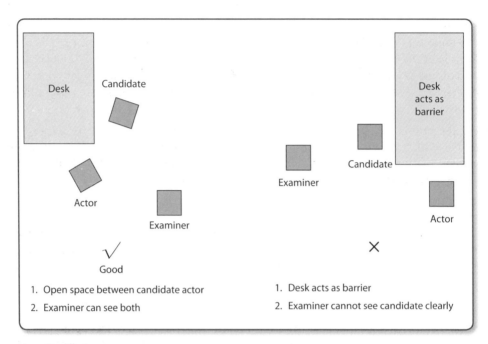

**Figure 3.1** Chair arrangement

communication with the patient and allow the examiner to see you demonstrate the non-verbal communication. You will then be advised, usually by the ring of a bell, that you can start reading the instructions. This bell also indicates the start of the 10 minutes, so after reading time and inviting the patient to enter the room, you will probably have nearer to 9 minutes to complete the task.

## Consultation skills

The consultations are simulated and you should remember that the actors have a brief and are playing a role. They will not tell you irrelevant information and you should therefore listen to and explore any clues an actor may give. This includes picking up emotional cues and addressing these – does the actor seem upset or anxious? If so, ask why.

Whilst the simulated consultations are obviously not real you should imagine that they are. Immerse yourself in the scenario and don't act – be yourself.

There is no single right way to consult, and your individuality should be encouraged. However, to help you consult effectively and gather all of the information it is important to consider a few core consultation skills in detail; with practice, you should be able to incorporate these into your natural consultation style.

### Active listening

Listening is a difficult and complex skill that involves much more than just hearing a patient's responses. The following skills and techniques are all included under the umbrella of 'active listening'.

**Listen**

The most important thing to remember to do is to listen. Candidates are often so focussed thinking of the next question to ask that they do not listen to the patient's answer and fail to respond to the patient's cues or emotion. This results in the patients having to repeat themselves and candidates failing to pick up on cues and being marked poorly.

Do not make the mistake of thinking that unless you are talking you are not earning marks. With practice you will realise that 10 minutes is plenty of time; if you can get the actor to talk for 2 minutes, they will have told you more or less everything in their brief (this should be the aim) and you will have scored highly.

**Open questions**

Open questions allow the patient to tell the story in a complete way. They prevent the 'stab in the dark' approach of closed questions and give you time to listen and think about the issues rather than just planning your next question.

Allow the patient to speak – your patients are actors playing a role to a set brief and the more opportunities you give them to speak the more information you will be given.

It will often take at least three open-ended questions to ascertain what is going on. Try to not give up and revert to doctor-centred closed questions if the patient is cagey – the actor may have been told not to give too much away initially. Open questions are much more helpful to gather reliable information. Whilst closed questions do have their role, they may be distorted by the practitioner's assumptions and can therefore cause misinterpretation of the case. Examples of open questions are:

**D:** How can I help you today?
**D:** Can you tell me a bit more about that?

**Reflecting back**

This is a useful tool for showing the patient (and examiner) that you have been listening and are interested in what they are saying. It can be very brief (it is not a full summary of what they have been saying) and it can link questions well.

**D:** You mentioned that work is stressful could you tell me a bit more about that?
**D:** You told me earlier that you had tried to give up smoking – could you tell me how that went?

**Empathy**

Empathy is being attentive, caring, providing support and showing you understand how the patient feels. It involves adapting your approach to a situation and examiners often mark candidates down for making empathetic statements but not matching these with their non-verbal approach. Non-verbal empathetic behaviour includes:

- Nodding your head.
- Leaning slightly forwards.
- Silence.
- Encouraging noises – umm, OK, yes.
- Facial expressions to reflect emotions (smile, grimace, sadness).

It is not enough to simply state: 'I know this must be very stressful for you' – you *must* *be sincere.*

### Silence

Silence is an excellent way of encouraging the patient to tell you what has been happening and any thoughts they have had. Try not to interrupt because the patient will fill the silence by giving you valuable information and clues.

Silence at the right time in a consultation is also an exceptionally powerful way of dealing with difficult, upsetting situations. Silence shows you are listening, that you understand the importance of what the patient is saying and that you are comfortable dealing with their emotion.

### Clarifying

Clarifying what a patient has said demonstrates that you have been listening to them and want to get to the bottom of the problem.

D:  You mentioned this started a long time ago – when exactly did things start getting difficult?

## Exploring ideas, concerns and expectations (ICE)

It is crucial to explore why a patient presented and what the patient is most worried about. The answers that a patient gives can define the consultation. Furthermore, any reassurance you may give to a patient can only be correctly directed if you understand the patients' concerns. Never assume you know what a patient is worried about – always ask.

Ideally ICE will be explored once the patient has given plenty of information and possibly dropped a cue. You should experiment with the way you ask the questions because this will impact on the answers you receive. This is demonstrated by the following examples:

D:  What do you think is going on?
P:  I don't know; that is why I have come to see you.
D:  Did you have any concerns?
P:  Of course I do –I want to know what is going on.
D:  What were you hoping I could do?
P:  Find out what is wrong with me!

This dialogue shows a clumsy way of exploring ICE and gains very little information. Each question should be altered to the situation, and it can be helpful to reflect what the patient has previously told you, for example:

D:  You have told me about this pain you have been having but do you have any particular thoughts about what could be causing it?
P:  Well, my mother had bowel cancer and I'm a bit worried that it could be that.

It is important to recognise if a patient has already expressed a concern because if asked again this simply demonstrates the doctor has not been listening. For example:

**P:**   I don't think all the stress at home can be helping things.

Later on:

**D:**   What do you think is causing your symptoms?

The doctor's unstructured method of questioning has shown a failure to listen actively. Instead, the following could be said:

**D:**   You mentioned before that you thought stress at home was causing your symptoms but did you have any other thoughts?

As ever, practice makes perfect – experiment with different phrases you feel comfortable with until you feel confident.

## Signposting

Signposting allows you to keep control of the consultation, progress smoothly from one section to another and indicate a change in direction. It allows the patient (and the examiner) to know where you are going (and why). It is a very useful technique to allow you to move from open to closed questions and also to draw a line underneath something and move on (e.g. result-giving, a complaint, frustrations). For example:

**D:**   Thank you for telling me about the pain – would you mind if I asked you a few specific questions?
**D:**   I can really understand why you are so frustrated and I completely agree that we need to investigate why this has happened but perhaps we can now talk about what we can do to improve the situation.
**D:**   I can reassure you that your tests are entirely normal but I appreciate you still have the pain. Could we spend a moment thinking about what could be done to improve your symptoms?

## Summarising

Summarising within a consultation is a skill that is difficult to perfect. Done properly, this is an excellent method to show that you have understood and remembered the key points of the consultation and explored the patient's ideas, concerns and expectations. It can also be used if you feel the consultation has become unstructured and when you want to check with the patient that nothing has been missed. It may also allow you the opportunity to revisit cues that have not been explored.

It is not appropriate in every consultation but is a good tool to use if you feel you have not quite understood what is going on yourself. An example of how to begin summarising would be:

**D:**   Would you mind if I just recap some of the things we have been talking about so you can tell me if I have missed anything?

## Safety netting

Safety netting is the way GPs deal with uncertainty. In simple terms it is explaining to the patient what they should look out for, i.e. what symptoms may be of concern and ensuring that they know your door is open for them to come back. The last thing a GP would want is for a patient to stay at home with worsening symptoms just because the GP had given reassurance earlier that day.

## Organising follow-up

Organising follow-up can be an excellent way of scoring extra marks. Try to reflect back on what you have been told. If the patient is busy at home or work you can organise telephone follow-up. If they work long hours they may be able to have an evening or Saturday morning appointment.

**D:**  I would like to see you again to see how things are going but I know work is busy so perhaps a telephone appointment would be easiest for you.

## Key points

- Don't act – be yourself.
- There is no one right way to consult.
- Listen and allow the patient to talk.
- Use open questions.
- Explore ICE.

# Interpreting the candidate's instructions and case brief

The candidate's brief can provide important information. Sometimes it will be short and provide few clues as to the nature of the consultation, whilst other instances will be much longer. We have tried to reflect this variability in the practice cases in Chapter 4.

Try to read the brief carefully so you don't need to keep referring back to it during the consultation. You can often predict what the case may involve before the patient enters the room. The following instructions are the same for all of the cases, but make sure you read the setting i.e. hospital or general practice.

> In this exercise you will be consulted by a patient in an acute hospital setting. The role of the patient will be taken by someone not directly involved in the assessment process, although their written evaluation of your performance may be used for reference in the final discussions.
>
> You have 10 minutes to complete this exercise which includes reading time. When you are ready please invite the patient into the room.

Or alternatively:

> In this exercise you will be consulted by a patient in a general practice setting. The role of the patient will be taken by someone not directly involved in the assessment process, although their written evaluation of your performance may be used for reference in the final discussions.
>
> You have 10 minutes to complete this exercise which includes reading time. When you are ready please invite the patient into the room.

National Recruitment Office for General Practice Training. Stage 3 Example Scenarios.  http://www. gprecruitment.org.uk/downloads/Stage%203%20examples%202011.pdf.

Spend a moment reading the instructions carefully and have a quick think about what the case may involve, as in the following three examples.

## Case 1

You are working as an FY2 doctor in general practice. Mrs Mary Jones, aged 60 years, previously saw your colleague. The consultation notes and subsequent investigation results are below.

Colicky generalised abdominal pain with bloating. Intermittent constipation and diarrhoea. Bloods: full blood count and liver function tests normal. Colonoscopy: good views obtained from rectum to caecum, normal mucosa throughout.

Your immediate thoughts should be that the likely diagnosis is irritable bowel syndrome and the consultation could involve:

- Establishing the patient's prior knowledge.
- Explaining results.
- Exploring ideas and concerns (e.g. did the patient think she had cancer?).
- Management of irritable bowel syndrome and discussing triggers (why now – stress?).
- Discussion of solutions and treatments.

## Case 2

You are a junior doctor working in clinic.

Mrs Jones, a 64-year-old patient, returns for her endoscopy result. The report states:

Normal oesophagus, mild antral gastritis only. CLO test positive. (NB The CLO test looks for presence of *Helicobacter pylori*.)

Your immediate thoughts should be that the likely diagnosis is Helicobacter infection and gastritis, and the consultation could involve:

- Establishing the patient's prior knowledge.
- Explaining investigation results (using lay terms and analogies, and checking understanding).
- Exploring ideas, concerns and expectations.
- Organising follow up and safety net processes.

## Case 3

You are a GP. Mrs Jameson has booked to see you. She had a biopsy of a lesion on her leg in the surgery 3 weeks ago. The lesion was thought to be benign but a biopsy was taken as the diagnosis was unclear. Unfortunately, the laboratory has lost the results and this means that you will have to repeat the biopsy.

Your immediate thoughts should concern the following:

- Breaking bad news (lost results).
- Dealing with an angry, frustrated patient.
- Exploring ideas, concerns and expectations.

# Specific situations

## Consultations with patients

There are situations that many candidates struggle to deal with. These difficult themes are briefly discussed below, to demonstrate methods of approaching them.

### Giving results

Doctors are taught to explore the patient's prior knowledge before giving investigation results. This sometimes leads to awkward situations in time-pressured examinations because the candidate realises that the case is about giving the results and exploring the issues around that and it is not about retaking the entire history. Equally if a candidate just says: *could you tell me a bit about what has been going on?* He or she may get the response: *is it not in the notes? I have just come to get my results.* Think of a phrase you feel comfortable using to start off such a consultation. For example:

**P:**  Hello, I've just come in to get my blood test results.
**D:**  Certainly, I have got your notes and results but it would be helpful if you could briefly tell me what has been going on, and what led you to have these tests.

### Dealing with a complaint or an angry patient

Candidates are concerned about admitting mistakes or blaming colleagues and as a result can seem defensive. This is the wrong approach and will make the consultation more difficult than it needs to be.

Allow the patient to vocalise their concerns, acknowledge that they are upset, and apologise for any hurt or stress caused (**Box 1**). Try to avoid getting into a debate about whether something has gone wrong. This may provoke an argument. For example:

**P:**  I have developed bedsores and have been left lying in urine for hours. The nurses are terrible and something needs to be done.
**D:**  I'm sorry you feel like that. I'm not really involved with the nursing care myself but I do know that the nurses are very busy and understaffed.

Whilst the doctor's response may be reasonable this sort of response will inflame the situation because the patient will not feel their concerns have been heard or taken seriously. A more measured response would be:

---

**Box 1: Dealing with anger**

- Stay calm, breath deeply and maintain an open posture.
- Actively listen and be interested in what has gone on.
- Do not be defensive.
- Don't raise your voice to match the patient's.
- Acknowledge that the patient is angry and apologise if something has gone wrong.
- Focus on what the patient needs and what can be done to help.
- Be aware of other emotions (e.g. sadness or fear) and explore these

D: I am really sorry that this has happened. It sounds absolutely terrible for you and what you are describing sounds very inadequate. We all strive to provide the best care possible but sometimes we fall short and need to look into why things have gone wrong to stop them happening again. Would you be able to tell me a bit more about what you have noticed?

In this case the doctor has acknowledged what has been said, apologised if any mistakes have occurred and has not given an already angry patient a reason to become more upset.

### Dealing with a patient who is requesting unnecessary tests, referrals or treatment

When a patient makes a request for something that you do not feel is appropriate, do not immediately refuse this or the consultation will be distorted by the patient's need to prove that the test or treatment is warranted. Instead you should try to get all of the history and explore the reasons for the request (remember: ICE).

P: I've got a really bad cold, my throat is sore and my nose is running so I just need a prescription for antibiotics.
D: A cold is actually a viral infection so antibiotics don't help.
P: Well, I have also been coughing and can hardly sleep.

This consultation is likely to continue in this dysfunctional manner. A different approach is not to address the antibiotic request until you have all of the information.

P: I've got a really bad cold, my throat is sore and my nose is running so I just need a prescription for antibiotics.
D: OK, could you tell me a bit more about what has been going on so I can work out the best treatment for you?

You can then take a full history, explore ICE, perform an examination (not in the selection centre) and toward the end of the consultation offer an explanation such as:

D: You mentioned earlier that you think you need antibiotics but after listening to what has been going on, and from the examination findings I think that this is a viral infection and so antibiotics won't do anything at all to help you. What you really need to do is ...

### Dealing with a delayed diagnosis

You should approach this case in the same way that you would when dealing with an angry patient. You may have to offer a chronological description of events and try to explain why the diagnosis wasn't made earlier. It can also be useful to offer to look in detail at the case, discuss it with the other doctors and agree to meet again to discuss what you have learnt. For example, for a patient who has recently been admitted to hospital with a gastrointestinal bleed caused by a peptic ulcer, and who had been seen 3 weeks before and started on omeprazole:

P: I've just come out of hospital doctor, it was horrible and could all have been avoided if you had picked up the problem earlier.
D: [after fully exploring what happened and what the patient's ideas are] I really can understand why you are frustrated. I'm so sorry to hear that you had to be admitted

to hospital and became so unwell. When you were seen a few weeks ago, the doctor started omeprazole because he thought you had a condition called gastritis. This is inflammation in the stomach. Omeprazole is actually also treatment for stomach ulcers. Your blood tests were normal at the time so there was no evidence that you had been bleeding at that point. This is the normal course of action because most patients improve and do not need any further tests, although if a patient's symptoms continue we would organise an endoscopy ...

### Dealing with a condition that you know nothing about

The simulation exercises don't specifically test clinical expertise but it is difficult to explain results or reassure a patient if you have no knowledge of a condition. Try not to be distracted by your knowledge level. Candidates who have a detailed knowledge of a condition often score less well than they should because they are keen to demonstrate their knowledge and forget to explore the underlying issues. Equally, candidates with limited knowledge can become flustered when they read the candidate's brief and consult less well than they otherwise would, for example:

**P:**  I am so worried about getting multiple sclerosis; the optician told me I have optic neuritis and I am hardly sleeping waiting to see the neurologist.

**D:**  I can understand why you are worried, it must be very stressful for you but actually only about 1 in 4 patients with optic neuritis go on to be diagnosed with multiple sclerosis. There are lots of other causes such as lupus, diabetes, viral infections ...

Whilst this may well demonstrate excellent knowledge the doctor's urge to display this has meant that he has failed to communicate clearly and the point has been missed. Imagine if you knew nothing about optic neuritis.

**P:**  I am so worried about getting multiple sclerosis; the optician told me I have optic neuritis and I am hardly sleeping waiting to see the neurologist.

**D:**  I am sure it is extremely stressful for you. Would you mind telling me a little bit about what has been going on?

**P:**  My sight started to get blurred on the left side and then it seemed to ache when I moved my eye so I panicked a bit and went to eye casualty. It is completely better now but they told me I had optic neuritis and that I needed to see a neurologist. I have been reading about it on the internet, I probably shouldn't have because it has been so scary.

**D:**  You mentioned that you are worried about multiple sclerosis – what sort of things have you been reading?

And so on. At some point the doctor may establish the patient is a single mother and is worried about how she would cope with multiple sclerosis, or that she has been referred to the neurologist but has not yet received an appointment. In this way, having little knowledge is not a hindrance. Also, never forget that the actor will have done this case hundreds of times already and will probably know more about it that you.

Be honest if you have no idea what the problem is, as you would be in everyday practice. It is well worth thinking about a phrase to explain that you are a bit out of your depth and need to get advice. Examples of such phrases are:

**D:**  I don't have a great deal of experience dealing with optic neuritis myself and I can appreciate it is frustrating waiting to see the neurologist. Would you like me to contact the neurology department to see if your appointment could be expedited?

**D:** I don't have a great deal of experience dealing with optic neuritis myself. Would it be possible for us to meet again in a couple of days, or for me to telephone you, and in the meantime I can talk to the neurologist and find out much more information for you.

## Consultations with a patient's relative

The communication skills being assessed are the same in all three exercises, although the focus and type of case will vary slightly. To help you tackle the sort of cases which often come up, specific situations and related background knowledge are given here.

### When a patient's relative is refusing help at home or a nursing home placement

- What is happening at home? What are the problems?
- What does the relative think should be done?
- What does the patient think and why are they refusing help?
- Empathise and acknowledge impact on relatives or carers lives as these can be extremely stressful situations for relatives.
- Try to come up with a solution – multidisciplinary team meeting, family meeting, etc.
- Explain capacity in lay terms (**Box 2**).
- You may need to be aware of funding rules (**Box 3**).

### When a relative thinks that a family member has dementia

- What has been going on? Ask for specific examples.
- What is the situation at home – living alone, friends or family close?
- Specifically ask about red flags:
  - Does the gas get left on?
  - Does the front door get left open?
  - Is there a risk of abuse or neglect?
- Explain dementia is a possibility but there are other conditions (i.e. depression) which mimic this.
- Try to come up with a solution that will provide an opportunity to assess the patient.
- If appropriate, consider mentioning lasting power of attorney (**Box 4**).

### Confidentiality

Candidates are often concerned about confidentiality. In most cases this doesn't arise as an issue, but the following guidelines should assist:

1. You can talk about a patient with a relative. However, unless it is specifically stated (in the candidate's brief) that you have their consent, avoid divulging information that you have been provided in the candidate's brief (i.e. their notes).

2. If you are being asked for sensitive information about a patient and you do not have the patient's consent, explain this and offer to talk in general terms, as appropriate to the case (see the Fraser competence example in Box 5, p. 72).

## Box 2 Capacity

- Understand the decision to be made and the consequences of that decision.
- Retain the information for long enough to make that decision.
- Way up the pros and cons of a decision.
- Communicate that decision.

There are five key principles in the Mental Health Act (cited by way of example as the act covers England and Wales only).

- Every adult has the right to make his or her own decisions and must be assumed to have the capacity to make them unless it is proved otherwise.
- A person must be given all practicable help before anyone treats them as not being able to make their own decisions.
- Just because an individual makes what might be seen as an unwise decision, they should not be treated as lacking capacity to make that decision.
- Anything done or any decision made on behalf of a person who lacks capacity must be done in their best interests.
- Anything done for or on behalf of a person who lacks capacity should be the least restrictive of their basic rights and freedoms.

Mental Health Act 2007. http://www.legislation.gov.uk/ukpga/2007/12/pdfs/ukpga_20070012_en.pdf.

## Box 3 Continuing care

In England and Wales, most patients have to fund their own care until they have reached a low threshold of capital (currently around £13,000). The patient's home will be taken into account (and hence it may need to be sold) unless it is also the sole home of their spouse (or certain other people, for example close relatives under 16).

A patient who meets specific ongoing medical care needs may be eligible for non-means tested funding of ongoing costs (so families are very keen to be granted 'continuing care').

To be eligible for continuing care the patient needs to have to have a complex medical condition that requires a great deal of care, support and usually specialised nursing care. A patient approaching the end of their life is also likely to be eligible, especially if they have a terminal condition and are rapidly deteriorating.

## Box 4 Power of attorney

A power of attorney is a legal document that allows a person to appoint someone else to manage his or her affairs in the event that he or she loses capacity to make decisions in the future. A power of attorney can include healthcare decisions. It has to be set up at a time when the patient has capacity.

## Confidentiality and the driving and vehicle licensing agency (DVLA)

There are a few occasions where it is necessary to disclose confidential information in the public interest. In the case of driving restrictions:

- A driver is legally required to inform the DVLA about any condition affecting ability to drive.
- If a driver refuses to accept the diagnosis of such a condition, a second opinion should be sought.
- If a patient continues to drive when the patient is not fit to do so, you should try to persuade the patient to stop.
- If you cannot persuade the patient to stop you should contact the DVLA immediately and speak to a medical advisor.
- Ideally you should inform the patient that you are going to call the DVLA and inform the patient in writing once you have done so.

## Request to amend medical records

Doctors have a legal duty to keep accurate, up-to-date medical records and patients have a right to ask for them to be amended. However, only factual errors should be amended, not professional opinions. It is not appropriate to delete records which a patient may feel will harm their employment prospects or insurance premiums. If in doubt, you can explain that these are difficult legal issues and speak to your medical defence organisation for advice.

## The relative who doesn't want the patient to know the diagnosis

The legal position is to act in the patient's best interests and do no harm. Try not to rush in to giving advice or explanations but explore:

- What does the patient think the diagnosis is?
- Why does the relative not want the patient to know?
- What does the relative think the patient already thinks or knows?

You could discuss the following aspects:

- Patients usually know the diagnosis (even if they don't say so) and are often relieved to get it out in the open.
- It is extremely rare that a patient is not told the diagnosis (usually the reason for withholding the information is if it would seriously impact on their mental or physical health).
- Failure to inform the patient may deny him or her the chance to write a will, say goodbye, and make plans.
- It may make ongoing treatment difficult.

## A mother who found her daughter's contraceptive pill and is requesting information about her daughter's care

At 16 years of age, a young person can be presumed to have the capacity to consent. A young person under the age of 16 years may have the capacity to consent, depending on maturity and ability to understand what is involved and so this has to be assessed.

Be prepared to explain Fraser competence (**Box 5**) to her mother. Thinking about phrases in advance can be helpful.

> **Box 5: Fraser competence (formerly Gillick competence)**
>
> A doctor can proceed to give advice and treatment without informing parents, provided the following criteria are satisfied:
> - That the girl (although under the age of 16 years of age) will understand the advice
> - That the doctor cannot persuade her to inform her parents or allow the doctor to inform the parents that she is seeking contraceptive advice
> - That she is very likely to continue to have sexual intercourse with or without contraceptive treatment
> - That unless she receives contraceptive advice or treatment, her physical or mental health or both are likely to suffer
> - That her best interests require the doctor to give her contraceptive advice, treatment or both without parental consent

**D:**  As Claire's doctor I have a duty of confidentiality to her as I do to all of my patients. I can't therefore discuss any specific details of her medical care but I can explain the process that doctors go through in these situations.

**D:**  I realise that this must be very difficult and frustrating for you.

**D:**  When dealing with young people we always encourage them to discuss their care with their parents and we always have their best interests and safety in mind.

**D:**  In situations where young people feel unable to involve their family we do prescribe contraception if that is in their best interest.

## Consultations with (non-medical) healthcare professionals

This exercise tests your ability to communicate effectively with colleagues, value team members and problem solve effectively. The same communication skills that were discussed earlier in this chapter are once again being assessed. You are likely to be faced with situations or problems that you haven't previously experienced and you will be expected to offer advice or come up with a solution. The following types of cases often arise:

### A colleague wanting to discuss medical or personal issues

It is important to be empathetic and supportive but also to recognise professional boundaries. Demonstrate active listening: find out what is happening and what your colleague thinks should be done. Make suggestions and (depending on the situation) advise them to make an appointment to see their own GP. Offer to meet them again to see how things are going. Try not to offer a prescription, sick note, etc.

### Counselling colleagues

A colleague may wish to discuss a case, especially if it has affected him or her. Explore his concerns. Why was this case so stressful? Pick up on cues – is anything else going on? Has it brought back personal memories? For example, you might say: 'You seem particularly affected by this case, is there any specific reason why?' Empathise with the colleague.

**Dealing with underperforming colleagues**

Colleagues may wish to raise concerns about another healthcare professional.

- Explore – what are the concerns? What has happened?
- Think – has patient safety been put at risk or will it be in future?
- Reassure the colleague – whistleblowing is stressful and raising this issue is the right thing to do.
- Verbalise your thoughts (see the example below).

Remember that the GMC states: 'Act without delay if you have good reason to believe that you or a colleague may be putting patients at risk.'

When a colleague is underperforming you will need to make a judgment about what the most appropriate response is. This could range from a quiet chat at a convenient time to ensuring that your colleague stops working immediately (e.g. if intoxicated at work). Remember that your colleague may have a very reasonable explanation and may welcome the chance to unload. On the other hand, your questioning may be deemed is an unnecessary intrusion. You may find the following approach helpful in these situations:

1. Deal with immediate risk: approach the colleague and explain that patients are being put at risk. Advise cessation of work and ensure that the work is covered.

2. Get help: discuss with a senior colleague, e.g. a consultant or clinical director. If you don't feel that the senior colleague is dealing with the issue, it may need to go higher.

3. Support your colleague: there may be reasons for poor performance and support may be needed.

**Bullying, sexual harassment or racism at work**

Listen to your colleague and encourage him or her to be open and honest. Offer reassurance that there will be support, and that the behaviour experienced is completely unacceptable and needs to be dealt with, for example:

D: You are absolutely right to have raised this and I can understand why you are so upset by it.

D: Racism is completely unacceptable and we need to deal with this.

Do verbalise your thoughts. Candidates often have a lot of thoughts about what may be done, or what may be the underlying cause for a situation, but find it difficult to verbalise them when there is such limited information. One useful thing to remember is to 'think out loud' and verbalise your thoughts i.e.:

D: I think it is absolutely right of you to have raised concerns about Dr James. I wonder whether there is any reason that he has started to miss work and turn up late. He may need additional support but it certainly needs to be looked into because all of his colleagues are being put under pressure covering for him and at some point patient care may be put at risk.

# Chapter 4

# Simulated consultation exercises

This chapter provides 45 simulated consultation exercises. Each one sets out a short clinical scenario and provides a briefing for the exam candidate and for the actor who will play the part of a patient, a relative or a healthcare professional. For each consultation, a clinical scenario is described and where appropriate test results are included.

Simulated consultations with patients: p. 86

Simulated consultations with relatives: p. 101

Simulated consultations with healthcare professionals: p. 116

For each of the exercises, Chapter 5 gives a transcribed example of a well-performed consultation.

# Patient scenario 1

## Candidate instructions

In this exercise you will be consulted by a patient in an acute hospital setting.

**Your task: you have a total of 10 minutes (including reading time) to complete this exercise. When you are ready to begin the consultation, please invite the patient to enter the room.**

You are an FY2 doctor working on an acute medical ward. A staff nurse on your ward asks you to see a patient before he is discharged. Mr Ward is a 68-year-old man who has been newly diagnosed with chronic obstructive pulmonary disease (COPD), after being admitted with pneumonia that was successfully treated. He has been prescribed inhalers and is due for follow-up by community COPD nurses and the chest clinic.

## Actor instructions

You are Mr Ward, a 65-year-old butcher who has been smoking for 40 years. You were admitted with a chest infection and have been diagnosed with something called COPD. You don't really understand what this is but you know that you have to use inhalers.

Your father died in pain at the age of 70 with lung cancer, and you are understandably worried that because of your smoking history and your new diagnosis of COPD it is inevitable that you will also get lung cancer.

You would like to give up smoking, but in many ways you think that any changes you make now are too little too late. Is it really worth you giving up? You tried patches a few years ago but you only managed to stop for a few months.

You live with your wife who has very poor mobility as a result of a diabetic foot ulcer. You have been breathless for a few months and have been having difficulty walking to the shops. You are worried about this getting worse and want to know how to make sure your condition improves or at least remains stable.

You have been under a great deal of stress because your wife is less able to do chores around the house and you would gladly welcome some help at home.

This case tests a candidate's ability to explain a diagnosis, explore the underlying concerns (lung cancer, inability to cope at home) and a good candidate should also explore smoking cessation.

## General manner

Friendly but a bit confused by everything.

## Patient scenario 2

### Candidate instructions

In this exercise you will be consulted by a patient in a GP setting.

**Your task: you have a total of 10 minutes (including reading time) to complete this exercise. When you are ready to begin the consultation, please invite the patient to enter the room.**

You are a GP working in a practice. Your next patient is Mr Xavi, a 58-year-old man who has come in to discuss his blood test results. He was seen in the rapid access chest pain clinic 1 month ago, where resting and exercise ECGs were both normal. It was decided then that he was suffering from non-cardiac chest pain, but he was advised to see his GP to discuss his elevated lipid level. His cholesterol is 7.2 mmol/L (normal range 2–5 mmol/L) and his blood pressure is 140/87 mmHg.

### Actor instructions

You are a 58-year-old cleaner who has come to get your blood test results. You are extremely worried because you have been told they are abnormal. The last few weeks have been very stressful after you developed chest pain and attended the emergency department and subsequently the rapid access chest pain clinic. You had some 'heart tests' and were told that everything was fine, but you needed to see your GP about the results of the blood test.

You remain very concerned about the possibility of a heart attack despite reassurance that your chest pain was not a heart attack. You think that having high cholesterol will lead to a heart attack soon. Your excessive anxiety has probably developed because your next-door neighbour, who was younger than you (49 years old), died of a heart attack 3 months ago.

You live alone and are worried that something will happen to you and no one will be there to help. You are recently divorced from your wife and you have one son, who lives abroad.

This case requires the candidate to explain test results to a confused, anxious patient who seems convinced that they are going to have a heart attack. This needs to be addressed directly.

### General manner

A little confused, anxious and worried. Will be reassured by clear, calm explanation.

## Patient scenario 3

### Candidate instructions

In this exercise you will be consulted by a patient in a GP setting.

### Your task: you have 10 minutes to complete this exercise, which includes reading time. When you are ready, please invite the patient into the room.

Your next patient is a 23-year-old woman, Miss Yetton. She has asked to be seen regarding ongoing headaches. She was previously seen by another GP in the practice who arranged for a CT – this was normal. Neurological examination was also normal. The other GP thought that these headaches were tension headaches.

### Actor instructions

You are Miss Yetton, a 23-year-old student studying law. You have been getting headaches for the last 6 months and have been told by a different GP that these are tension headaches.

Your headache is mainly across your forehead and comes on every day. It is sometimes relieved by paracetamol and sleeping. You have no photophobia, neck stiffness, rashes, nausea or visual disturbance. Your headache is not worse in the morning but it is worse after sitting in front of a computer for several hours.

You have had a CT and were told that this was normal but you are still worried about a brain tumour, because you read one report on the internet stating that small tumours may not be picked up on CTs. You think you should be seen by a neurologist and would like an MRI. You want the headache to be cured and not just 'masked' by painkillers.

You live with other students and all of you are studying for your final exams. You have a job lined up for next year and are anxious that if you fail you will not be able to take up this position. You have been studying for 12 hours every day and you are not sleeping well as you feel very stressed about things.

This case deals with a request for investigations that are not required and the candidate's ability to get to the bottom of the issue, in this case stress and overworking. The diagnosis is tension headaches and a good candidate should establish the likely cause of this and discuss ways of reducing the symptoms.

### General manner

Irritated that there is no instant cure, but will be calmed if your concerns are addressed in a sensitive manner.

## Patient scenario 4

### Candidate instructions

In this exercise you will be consulted by a patient in a GP setting.

**Your task: you have 10 minutes to complete this exercise, which includes reading time. When you are ready, please invite the patient into the room.**

You are a GP working in a practice. Your next patient is Mr Cavanagh, who has come to see you about pain in his left elbow. This has previously been diagnosed as tennis elbow and he has already been referred for physiotherapy.

Other treatment options, if asked are:

1. Topical analgesia.
2. Physiotherapy.
3. Oral analgesia – paracetamol, ibuprofen (unless contraindicated), codeine, tramadol, etc.
4. Steroid injection.

### Actor instructions

You are Mr Cavanagh, a 35-year-old builder who has been diagnosed with tennis elbow. You agree that this is the correct diagnosis, having read about it on the internet, but you are frustrated by the continued pain. You are waiting to start physiotherapy in 4 weeks' time and have been taking regular paracetamol, which has not been helping with the pain. You are very concerned as this has been affecting your work and, because you are self-employed, you cannot take time off.

You are worried that physiotherapy may not help and if you are unable to work you cannot earn. You have a wife and a 2-year-old baby and your income has been affected by the financial crisis, with much less building work available at the moment. You are struggling to cope with paying bills as your wife is looking after your child at home.

This case is designed to see how well a candidate acknowledges the way illness impacts on a patient's life. The candidate will hopefully establish the fact you are self-employed and any absence from work will have huge implications on your already-stretched finances. This is a fairly simple case but requires the candidate to approach it holistically and not simply focus on pain management.

### General manner

Anxious for a solution and may get frustrated if issues and concerns are not addressed.

## Patient scenario 5

### Candidate instructions

In this exercise you will be consulted by a patient in a hospital setting.

**Your task: you have a total of 10 minutes (including reading time) to complete this exercise. When you are ready to begin the consultation, please invite the patient to enter the room.**

You are a rheumatology FY2 and are covering the outpatient clinic while your consultant is away. He has given you instructions not to start new treatments, but to manage the patients' symptoms until he returns.

Your next patient, Mrs Nicholls, is a 38-year-old woman newly diagnosed with rheumatoid arthritis (serum RA positive and anti-CCP antibody positive). You need to tell the patient the diagnosis.

### Actor instructions

You are Mrs Nicholls, a 38-year-old violinist. You have come to clinic today to find out the results of your tests. You were referred to the clinic by your GP because you started getting pain and stiffness in your hands. This is worse in the morning and seems to improve throughout the day, but you still find it difficult to play the violin. You were seen a few weeks ago and the consultant thought it could be rheumatoid arthritis but wanted to do a few more tests.

You are devastated when you hear the news that you have rheumatoid arthritis. You had suspected it but were holding out hope for an alternative explanation for your symptoms. Your pain is well controlled with paracetamol and ibuprofen at the moment.

You play the violin professionally and are very worried that you will not be able to do this anymore. You are also worried about your 11-year-old daughter, and would like to know whether she may develop it in the future. Your aunt had rheumatoid arthritis and ended up being severely disfigured and disabled.

You have a supportive husband who earns enough to support you (as he is a banker) but you are worried about how he would feel if you ended up in a wheelchair like your aunt.

This case tests a candidate's ability to give bad news sensitively and explore the issues surrounding an illness or diagnosis.

### General manner

Anxious and upset.

# Patient scenario 6

## Candidate instructions

In this exercise you will be consulted by a patient in a GP setting.

**Your task: you have a total of 10 minutes (including reading time) to complete this exercise. When you are ready to begin the consultation, please invite the patient to enter the room.**

Mrs Jameson has booked to see you. She had a biopsy of a lesion on her leg in the surgery 3 weeks ago. The lesion was initially thought to be benign, but the biopsy was taken as the diagnosis was unclear. Unfortunately, the laboratory has lost the sample and this means that you will have to repeat the biopsy.

## Actor instructions

You are Mrs Jameson, a 56-year-old cleaner. You contacted the surgery yesterday to get the results of the biopsy taken from your leg, but were told that the sample has been lost. You are extremely angry and upset. How can such a mistake happen? Who is to blame?

You are the main breadwinner at home and are self-employed, so taking time off work to have a repeat biopsy costs you money. You are also extremely worried about cancer. Your mother died of melanoma and you are extremely worried that this lesion is malignant. You have hardly slept for the past few weeks waiting for these results and are incredibly upset that they have been lost.

You calm down a little if the doctor seems to understand your frustrations and tries to come up with some solutions to help you. You also respond well to reassurances that skin cancer at this point is unlikely.

This case aims to test a candidate's ability to calm down an angry patient, acknowledge her concerns and try to come up with a reasonable solution.

## General manner

Upset, angry and frustrated.

## Patient scenario 7

### Candidate instructions

In this exercise you will be consulted by a patient in a GP setting.

**Your task: you have 10 minutes to complete this exercise, which includes reading time. When you are ready, please invite the patient into the room.**

You are working as an FY2 doctor in general practice. Mrs Louise Armstrong is a 60-year-old woman who has recently had tests after seeing your colleague 1 month ago. The consultation notes and subsequent investigation results are:

Colicky generalised abdominal pain with bloating. Intermittent constipation and diarrhoea.

Blood tests – full blood count, liver function tests – normal.

Colonoscopy – good views obtained from rectum to caecum, normal mucosa throughout.

### Actor instructions

You are Louise Armstrong, a 60-year-old woman who has been unwell over the past few months with abdominal pain, bloating and occasional diarrhoea. You were very worried that this was bowel cancer, especially when the GP said that you needed to have a colonoscopy.

You have come back to get the results. The hospital doctor doing the colonoscopy didn't say much but you got the impression that there wasn't a great deal wrong. Despite this, your symptoms continue.

You have been very stressed recently and think that the stress must be affecting you. Your mother is in a nursing home and they keep contacting you to ask you for things. Usually they are very minor requests – for example asking you to buy her a new pair of tights, but you always feel worried that something is seriously wrong when they leave messages asking for you to call back.

You work as a teacher and things at school are very busy at the moment. You have an inspector's report coming up and are feeling under pressure.

This case tests the ability of candidates to give results, explore concerns and establish what could be causing your symptoms.

### General manner

Calm – relieved to be given the all clear but worried that your symptoms will continue.

# Patient scenario 8

## Candidate instructions

In this exercise you will be consulted by a patient in a GP setting.

**Your task: you have 10 minutes to complete this exercise, which includes reading time. When you are ready, please invite the patient into the room.**

Mrs White has booked in to see you during your morning surgery. You see from the notes that she has recently been diagnosed with deep vein thrombosis (DVT). Her combined oral contraceptive pill was stopped by the hospital and a thrombophilia screen was performed (which came back normal). She has been discharged and advised to continue warfarin for 3 months.

## Actor instructions

You are Mrs White, a 32-year-old woman who developed a swollen painful right leg a couple of weeks ago. You attended the emergency department and were admitted to hospital the same day, where you were diagnosed with DVT. You have no idea how or why this happened and you have been quite shaken by the whole experience. You consider yourself fit and healthy and have in fact been training to run the London Marathon.

You have booked in to see the doctor for a few reasons. You want to know exactly what DVT is and why you developed it. You would also ideally like to stop the warfarin – going to hospital every week for blood tests is so disruptive and your boss (you work in advertising) isn't at all happy. You are meant to be going away on business next week and will be away for 2 weeks. You also want to know why they told you to stop taking the pill and when you can start retraining for the marathon.

This case tests a candidate's ability to explain a simple diagnosis (DVT), explain the importance of anticoagulation and understand the implications of the diagnosis and its treatment.

### General manner

Calm, but will push for answers if you feel your questions are being avoided.

## Patient scenario 9

### Candidate instructions

In this exercise you will be consulted by a patient in a GP setting.

**Your task: you have 10 minutes to complete this exercise, which includes reading time. When you are ready, please invite the patient into the room.**

Mr Medland has booked in to see you. He was seen 2 weeks ago by one of your colleagues, when he complained of suffering with fatigue. Blood tests were arranged and he was asked to come back 1 week after they were taken to discuss the results.

Full blood count, renal, liver and thyroid function are all within the normal range.

### Actor instructions

You are Mr Medland, a 55-year-old man who has been feeling exhausted for the past few months. You are constantly fatigued and even when you sleep for 8 hours you still feel very tired. You went to see the doctor a few weeks ago because you thought there must be some underlying cause and blood tests were organised.

You work as a store assistant in a DIY shop, but you also took on a second job last year working in the local petrol station in the evenings. You are happily married but your wife was made redundant last year (hence the need for your second job) and this has put a strain on the relationship. You think she should do more to help you look after your father, who had a stroke last year. Although he still lives at home independently he tends to call every day and you end up visiting him very often because he is so lonely. By the time you get home you are absolutely exhausted and extremely stressed.

Your wife was very keen for you to visit the doctors. She thinks that there must be something wrong with your liver because you drink so much (five or six pints a night) so you are relieved to hear that your liver tests are fine.

This case examines a candidate's ability to explore the issues underlying a presentation. It is not simply a case of explaining normal investigation results.

### General manner

Calm, tired and hoping for an easily rectifiable problem.

# Patient scenario 10

## Candidate instructions

In this exercise you will be consulted by a patient in a GP setting.

**Your task: you have 10 minutes to complete this exercise, which includes reading time. When you are ready, please invite the patient into the room.**

Mr Livesey, 27-years-old, has booked in to see you. He is newly registered and you don't have any medical notes for him.

## Actor instructions

You have booked in to see the doctor at the request of your girlfriend who thinks you need help. You have recently left the Army after having done tours of both Iraq and Afghanistan. Whilst you had never intended to stay in the Army for long, your resignation was precipitated by the death of one of the soldiers under your command during your last tour in Afghanistan. He was killed by a roadside bomb and both you and the medic in your troop attended to him before he was evacuated.

You have been haunted by the memories of this event. You struggle to sleep and wake during the middle of the night with vivid images of the incident. You also feel extremely guilty that you were unable to lead your entire troop through the tour safely. You had some counselling when you got back home initially, and just got on with your job. Now you find there is no one to talk to who understands (you have much less contact with your military friends now) and the monotony of life outside the Army gives you so much time to think about things.

You are currently working in the city doing recruitment and have moved in with your girlfriend. She gets frustrated that you aren't getting help and is angry that you keep saying that things will settle down.

This case examines a candidate's ability to deal with a difficult problem in a patient who has been reluctant to seek help and is somewhat ashamed for needing help.

### General manner

Embarrassed because you feel like you are wasting the doctor's time.

# Patient scenario 11

## Candidate instructions
In this exercise you will be consulted by a patient in a GP setting.

### Your task: you have 10 minutes to complete this exercise, which includes reading time. When you are ready, please invite the patient into the room.
Mrs Jones, 68 years old, was last seen 6 months ago with left knee pain. She was advised then about weight loss and quadriceps strengthening exercises.

## Actor instructions
You are Mary Jones – a 68-year-old hairdresser. You are very worried because over the last 3 months you have lost half a stone in weight and have noticed that you have been having rather erratic bowel motions – usually looser than normal. You have also noticed blood in your motions. You saw an advert on television saying that this may be a sign of bowel cancer but have really delayed seeing the doctor because you are very frightened of hospitals.

You have spent the past few weeks on the internet and cannot bear the thought of having a colonoscopy. It sounds so degrading and painful. Your husband died suddenly a few years ago. He was rushed to hospital but sadly died in the emergency department. Since this point hospitals have given you a bad feeling and you didn't even manage to visit your sister in hospital when she was ill last year.

You are very concerned about the chance that you may have cancer and also about the possible investigations and treatment.

This case is designed to test a candidate's ability to listen to an anxious patient and reassure her that her concerns regarding investigations will be listened to.

### General manner
Very anxious.

# Patient scenario 12

## Candidate instructions

In this exercise you will be consulted by a patient in a GP setting.

## Your task: you have 10 minutes to complete this exercise, which includes reading time. When you are ready, please invite the patient into the room.

Sophie Blackmore is a 19-year-old girl who is currently 20 weeks pregnant. Her pregnancy is going well so far, although she has recently been treated for a lower respiratory tract infection with antibiotics.

## Actor instructions

You are Sophie; you are 19 years old and are currently 20 weeks pregnant. You became pregnant unexpectedly and you have since broken up with your boyfriend. He doesn't really want anything to do with the pregnancy and would have preferred you to have ended the pregnancy. Now the initial shock has gone you are excited about becoming a mother and are trying to get everything sorted out.

You currently live with your mother and siblings but have applied for housing yourself (there wouldn't be enough room at your mum's and you want to be independent). You have been offered a nice flat about 4 miles away from your mother's house, but you don't want to move this far away. You think that you'll really need her help once the baby is born. Being pregnant, you are already prioritised for housing but really want to live near your mother. You spoke to the Citizens Advice bureau and they advised that this might be possible if you get a letter from the GP explaining that you have medical problems.

You grew up in this area and have lots of friends. Two of your friends are already mothers and have been giving you advice. You currently smoke and have been trying to cut down but find it very hard.

This case is designed to test the candidate's ability to deal with an unreasonable request from a patient whilst maintaining a good rapport and exploring other ways to deal with the problem.

### General manner

Calm, really want to be near to your mother and don't think you could cope alone so fairly pushy for the letter.

# Patient scenario 13

## Candidate instructions

In this exercise you will be consulted by a patient in a GP setting.

## Your task: you have 10 minutes to complete this exercise, which includes reading time. When you are ready, please invite the patient into the room.

Miss Carter, 35 years old, has booked in to see you. She has recently been seen in eye casualty – the discharge note is given below.

Gradual onset of reduced vision in the left eye lasting 18 hours, but is now improving. Reduced pain accompanied by mild pain with eye movements. On examination, diagnosed with left eye optic neuritis. Will need further investigations and follow-up with neurologists. MRI arranged and neurology outpatient appointment requested.

## Actor instructions

You are Sarah Carter, a 35-year-old sales manager. You had a shock last week when you noticed the vision in your left eye becoming blurred. You went to eye casualty and were told it was optic neuritis. You are waiting for an MRI (next week) and also to see the neurologists (although you haven't heard anything about this appointment yet).

Since your visit to eye casualty your vision has improved, but you have been looking on the internet and have been really scared by what you have read. You think you have multiple sclerosis and will gradually lose your function. You have a 3-year-old son and are a single parent and you are very worried about how you will cope with any disability.

You can't stand the wait for the results and for the appointment with the neurologist. You are not sleeping and have no appetite. You haven't told anyone because you don't want to worry people until the diagnosis is confirmed.

Ideally you would like to hear good news (although you know the GP can't give you that) but you want the MRI and neurology appointment to be expedited.

This case explores a candidate's ability to communicate with an anxious patient when a diagnosis is unclear and complete reassurance cannot be given.

### General manner

Shocked, anxious and upset.

# Patient scenario 14

## Candidate instructions

In this exercise you will be consulted by a patient in a hospital setting.

## Your task: you have 10 minutes to complete this exercise, which includes reading time. When you are ready, please invite the patient into the room.

Miss Jackson, 26 years old, has asked to see you. She was admitted to the gastroenterology ward with a severe exacerbation of ulcerative colitis last week and was informed by the consultant this morning that she if she doesn't improve she may need surgery to remove an inflammatory stricture.

## Actor instructions

You are Katy Jackson, a 26-year-old events manager. You were diagnosed with ulcerative colitis 2 years ago after you developed bloody diarrhoea. The diagnosis was an enormous shock but until recently your illness has been reasonably well-controlled with mesalazine. Two weeks ago you started to feel unwell and had bloody diarrhoea. You tried to ignore it initially, as there were so many other things going on in your life. But eventually you became so weak that you were admitted to hospital last week.

This couldn't have come at a worse time for you. Work is incredibly busy – you are meant to be hosting a huge event this weekend, something you have been working towards for months. You are also due to get married in 3 months' time.

The surgeon came to see you and advised you that surgery may be necessary if you fail to improve on medication. He mentioned the possibility of a stoma – you can't bear the thought of this. How can you get married with a stoma? You think your fiancé would hate it.

You haven't mentioned it before, because you didn't want your consultant to be cross with you, but lately you have started smoking again, are eating meals at irregular times and you have forgotten to take the odd mesalazine. Is that what has caused this relapse?

This case explores a candidate's ability to discuss potentially life-changing surgery, empathise with the patient's concerns and provide as much reassurance as possible.

### General manner

Upset and anxious.

# Patient scenario 15

## Candidate instructions

In this exercise you will be consulted by a patient in a GP setting.

## Your task: you have 10 minutes to complete this exercise, which includes reading time. When you are ready, please invite the patient into the room.

Mrs Miah, 34 years old, has booked into see you. She is currently pregnant and was last seen when she was referred to the local hospital for antenatal care.

## Actor instructions

You are Mrs Miah, a 34-year-old woman. You are currently 17 weeks pregnant and have been told by the hospital that your baby has Down syndrome. You had an amniocentesis last week because the ultrasound tests suggested that this was a possibility. You hadn't really thought about what you would do if the amniocentesis confirmed Down syndrome and the last week has been extremely difficult.

You already have two healthy children aged 5 and 12 years old and your husband thinks you should terminate the pregnancy. He thinks it would be unfair on your other children to have such a dependent sibling. You can't bear the thought of terminating the pregnancy. For a start, as a Muslim it is against your religious beliefs but also you are carrying this child and you want to keep it. You have spoken to your mother who is also keen that you go through with the pregnancy because of your beliefs. Now you really wish you hadn't had the amniocentesis, because then you wouldn't be having these arguments.

You have done a bit of reading about Down syndrome and know there is a large variability of severity and that there is a risk of physical problems also. You think you can cope with this but are worried that your husband will always resent you for keeping the child.

You would be keen to get information and find out about local support groups. Most of all you just came to inform the GP and see if he or she has any suggestions.

This case is about a complex family situation requiring the candidate to respond in a sensitive and empathetic manner. The candidate should remain impartial and listen to the patient's concerns.

### General manner

Calm but looking for help and reassurance.

## Relative scenario 1

### Candidate instructions

In this exercise, you will be consulted by a patient's relative in a GP setting.

**Your task: you have a total of 10 minutes (including reading time) to complete this exercise. When you are ready please invite the relative to enter the room.**

You are an FY2 working in general practice. The wife of Mr Nigel Heath (66 years old) has booked to see you. Notes on his last two consultations are below. Mr Heath has given written consent for you to be able to discuss his medical records with his wife.

### December 2012

Persistent loose stools with bloating and weight loss. Previously assessed with bloods and colonoscopy – all normal. Refer to gastroenterology for opinion.

### January 2012

Colicky abdominal pain and excess wind eased by defecation. No weight loss. Stools generally looser than normal. Full blood count, urea and electrolytes, liver function tests and erythrocyte sedimentation rate – normal. Colonoscopy, good views obtained – normal investigation. Impression: diarrhoea-predominant irritable bowel syndrome.

### Actor instructions

Your husband has recently been diagnosed with coeliac disease. Since stopping all gluten his symptoms have resolved, he feels much better and has started to gain weight again. Before this diagnosis he was always bloated, felt tired and lethargic and had to pass wind frequently.

He saw the GP earlier in the year with the symptoms and was advised that he had irritable bowel syndrome. You know the doctor organised blood tests and a colonoscopy and can't believe it wasn't picked up at that point. If it had been, you would have been spared months of worry and, moreover, your husband would have been spared months of abdominal pain.

You are both retired and finances are tight. The hospital doctors gave your husband a prescription for some gluten-free bread but it was really tasteless and so you have been forced to buy branded products from the supermarket. It is so hard trying to exclude gluten from his diet and you don't know where to turn for help.

This case tests a candidate's ability to deal with an upset and angry relative in a difficult situation where blame is being apportioned.

### General manner

Initially angry. If the doctor empathises and explores your concerns you will calm down. Equally, if the doctor becomes very defensive you will find this very frustrating.

## Relative scenario 2

### Candidate instructions

In this exercise, you will be consulted by a patient's relative in a GP setting.

**Your task: you have a total of 10 minutes (including reading time) to complete this exercise. When you are ready to begin the consultation, please invite the relative to enter the room.**

You are an FY2 doctor working in general practice. Toby Young is a 42-year-old man who asks to speak to you regarding his father Jonathan Young (68 years old). You have not met his father before and the notes show that he was last seen 4 years ago with a chest infection. You have not been given consent to discuss his father's medical records.

### Actor instructions

You are concerned that your father is getting dementia. You have seen a lot about this in the media recently and you think that he has probably been 'losing his marbles' for quite a while. He is very forgetful but, when challenged, denies this and refuses to talk about it. He was found by his granddaughter to be wandering in town early one morning and has run out of petrol three times in the last few months. He also calls you in the middle of the night, disorientated about the time; for example, in February he called to ask you what you were doing for Christmas.

You think that he is neglecting himself, because he is losing weight and looks scruffy. He has lived alone since your mother died of breast cancer 10 years ago. He used to play golf but seems to have lost interest in doing this recently. He is a non-smoker and enjoys a whisky at bedtime.

You have a family history of Alzheimer's disease – your grandmother (paternal side) also suffered from dementia and became very distressed towards the end of her life. She kept accusing the family of abusing her and eventually couldn't recognise anyone. You were only a teenager at the time but remember feeling very upset by this.

You are feeling very stressed because you could not possibly cope with looking after your father if he becomes more unwell. You are also very concerned that you will develop dementia, as there is such a strong history in your family. You have started to do mind puzzles and Sudoku because you have read that this can prevent cognitive decline.

This case tests a candidate's ability to take a collateral history, understand the stress upon a carer and come up with a sensible plan.

### General manner

Calm.

## Relative scenario 3

### Candidate instructions
In this exercise, you will be consulted by a patient's mother in a GP setting.

### Your task: you have a total of 10 minutes (including reading time) to complete this exercise. When you are ready to begin the consultation, please invite the relative to enter the room.
Tom's mother Amy, 34 years old, consults you. Tom is an 8-year-old boy with no recent consultations.

### Actor instructions
You have booked an appointment with the GP because you are worried about your son. Tom used to enjoy school and have lots of friends, but he now resists going to school and frequently complains of abdominal pain. You suspect this is an excuse as he never actually seems in pain and is easily distracted by toys and games. The school has asked to see you twice because Tom has hit other pupils, which is totally unlike him – he used to be so kind and friendly. Tom seems withdrawn at home but whenever you try to discuss things with him he says he is fine and rushes off to his room.

You wonder whether his change in behaviour could have anything to do with your marital breakup last year, but you think it is unlikely because he seemed fine at the time. You have recently started seeing someone else and Tom gets on well with him. Tom still sees his father, although much less frequently now because his father has recently had another child with his new partner. You had wondered whether he is being bullied at school and so have spoken to his teachers but they haven't noticed anything going on.

You are really distressed about not connecting with Tom. You don't really know how the GP can help but you have come for support and hope that the doctor can offer a few suggestions. You work in a bookshop while Tom is at school and are coping fairly well.

This case aims to test a candidate's ability to empathise, appreciate how difficult the situation is and discuss a case where no specific cause or solution may be found.

### General manner
Concerned.

# Relative scenario 4

### Candidate instructions

In this exercise, you will be consulted by a relative of a patient in a hospital setting.

## Your task: you have a total of 10 minutes (including reading time) to complete this exercise. When you are ready to begin the consultation, please invite the relative to enter the room.

You are a junior doctor working in a care of the elderly ward. The ward clerk calls you to tell you that the daughter of one of your patients is very angry and would like to speak to you.

### Actor instructions

You are Mrs Nicholls. Your mother is 82 years old and was admitted to hospital from her nursing home after she became incoherent, confused and kept falling over. She had numerous tests and was eventually diagnosed with a urine infection. She has improved and is now back to her normal self, but she found the whole experience horrendous.

You think that the nursing care your mother received during her stay in hospital has been terrible. She has developed a new pressure sore and you believe that this is because the nurses have not been turning her and looking after her skin. On two occasions you have found her covered in urine; your mother said she had asked for a bedpan but it didn't come in time. You have also visited her and found a cold tray of uneaten food out of her reach and have heard other patients on the ward shouting for help but being ignored by the nursing staff. The nurses never seem to be able to tell you any details of your mother's care and seem generally disinterested.

The experience has made your mother say that she is never going to come back to hospital again. You have found it extremely upsetting; your mother is such a kind and caring lady and seeing her treated with such a lack of dignity and respect is horrible.

You want something to be done and you don't want any cover up, or defence of the indefensible.

This case examines a candidate's ability to calm an angry relative making complaints about other members of your team. A good candidate should acknowledge the complaint and seriousness of the matter and without trying to mount any defence.

### General manner

Initially angry and upset, but can be calmed down by appropriate responses from the doctor.

# Relative scenario 5

## Candidate instructions

In this exercise you will be consulted by a patient's relative in a hospital setting.

**Your task: you have a total of 10 minutes (including reading time) to complete this exercise. When you are ready to begin the consultation, please invite the relative to enter the room.**

You are a paediatric FY2. James Lewis, a 7-year-old boy, was admitted with an exacerbation of his asthma and is due to be discharged. His mother Sandy has asked to speak to you.

## Actor instructions

You are Sandy, a 35-year-old woman who has one 7-year-old son, James. He has asthma, which is usually well controlled with inhalers: beclomethasone twice daily and salbutamol as required. He has only been admitted to hospital twice, once when he was 2 years old and again 6 months ago.

You divorced your husband Alex 2 years ago. Alex lives with his new girlfriend, who you think smokes in the house. He denies this whenever you confront him about it but it is obvious because James always comes home smelling of cigarette smoke. You feel Alex has never taken James' asthma seriously enough and has not been giving him his steroid inhalers. You presume this is why his breathing deteriorates every time he goes and stays with his father.

You would like the doctors to discuss with James his asthma and the importance of taking his inhalers. You want to know if there is anyone you can speak to regarding this, as you are very worried that something may happen to James if this issue is not addressed.

Your relationship with James' father was very bad for a few years; eventually you had an affair with one of your friends and this led to your marriage breakdown. You have now remarried and are much happier. Alex has joint custody of James and looks after him on alternate weekends. You do feel very guilty about the fact that you had an affair and you do not want to restrict Alex from seeing James. Unfortunately, you don't trust him to look after James properly and if things don't change you will have to stop him staying there.

This case tests a candidate's ability to sensitively deal with difficult family issues.

## General manner

Stressed and worried.

## Relative scenario 6

### Candidate instructions

In this exercise, you will be consulted by a patient's relative in a GP setting.

### Your task: you have a total of 10 minutes (including reading time) to complete this exercise. When you are ready to begin the consultation, please invite the relative to enter the room.

Mr Brown's daughter has booked an appointment to see you. Mr Brown has been diagnosed with inoperable bronchial carcinoma following an episode of haemoptysis. He was last seen in the surgery 4 months ago (see the consultation note, below). You have Mr Brown's written consent to discuss his medical records with his daughter.

Chronic cough – worse in the last few months, smoker (lifelong with a 40 pack year history). No weight loss or haemoptysis.

Chest examination: mild expiratory wheeze only.

Chest X-ray – normal

COPD is likely. Advised smoking cessation, trial of inhalers and to see the nurse for spirometry tests when his cough has improved.

### Actor instructions

You have booked to see the GP to discuss your father's recent diagnosis of lung cancer. You are shocked, upset and scared. You knew that he had a chronic cough and that he had seen the GP about this a few months ago. He then started to cough up blood and so you made him go to the emergency department. Since then, he was seen in the respiratory clinic and diagnosed with inoperable lung cancer. You think they are planning some form of treatment, maybe radiotherapy or chemotherapy.

You are wondering why he was not diagnosed when he saw the GP a few months ago. You can accept any reasonable explanation (although you will get cross if it seems the doctor is covering things up). If the doctor seems understanding and explains things well your frustrations will ease.

Most of all, you are upset and worried and wonder how he will cope at home. How can you care for him yourself? What help is available? You also help to care for your mother, who has rheumatoid arthritis, and you don't think you could manage being a carer for both of your parents.

This case deals with a potential delayed diagnosis when the care provided seems reasonable. It requires the candidate to be honest and open, explain what has happened and explore the relative's other concerns.

### General manner

Angry and concerned. You will calm down if your concerns are addressed.

# Relative scenario 7

## Candidate instructions

In this exercise, you will be consulted by a patient's relative in an acute hospital setting.

**Your task: you have a total of 10 minutes (including reading time) to complete this exercise. When you are ready to begin the consultation, please invite the relative to enter the room.**

You are an FY2 doctor working on an acute medical ward. A staff nurse on your ward asks you to see a patient's son. The patient is a 79-year-old female, Mrs Potter, who came in after having fallen at home, fracturing the neck of her femur.

During her hospital admission she has developed both a urinary tract infection and hospital-acquired pneumonia, but is now recovering well and is keen to go home.

## Actor instructions

You are Mike Potter, a 38-year-old accountant living in Somerset with your wife and 3 young children, who are 11, 8 and 3 years old. Your mother, Mrs Potter, was admitted 5 weeks ago with a fractured hip and during her admission became unwell with a urine infection and then pneumonia.

You suspected that she was not coping before the fall and now she is even weaker. You have been trying to persuade her to move into a residential home nearer to you for months, but she is stubborn and can't contemplate leaving her home. It seems to be her body, not her mind, that is failing her as she has no cognitive impairment. Despite this, she lives in a cluttered mess and she seems to neglect herself. Her GP arranged a social services visit but she refused any help. Last year she still seemed fine and would go out to get her haircut, meet her friends and socialise, but lately she just stays at home watching television and getting weaker and weaker.

You don't think it is safe for her to go home. You thought this admission would give the social workers a chance to move her into a residential home, so you were shocked when the nurse told you she may be discharged next week. Has anyone done a proper assessment? You think it should be obvious that she can't cope and worry that she is being discharged prematurely. You have already taken quite a lot of time off work to get to London to see her and won't be able to stay with her when she is discharged.

This case tests a candidate's ability to establish a relative's concerns and address them, whilst dealing with the capacity of the patient to make her own decisions.

### General manner

Concerned but calm.

## Relative scenario 8

### Candidate instructions

In this exercise, you will be consulted by a patient's relative in an acute hospital setting.

**Your task: you have a total of 10 minutes (including reading time) to complete this exercise. When you are ready to begin the consultation, please invite the relative to enter the room.**

You are an FY2 doctor working in paediatrics. Tom (16 years old) was admitted last night after being brought to the emergency department following a drinks and drug binge. His mother, Mrs Martin, has booked in to see you.

### Actor instructions

You are Mrs Martin. Your 16-year-old son, Tom, was taken to the emergency department by ambulance last night after he collapsed at a friend's party. He was drunk and had used cocaine. You are so relieved that he is OK, but are absolutely devastated by the fact he has taken drugs. You knew he drank beer with friends and thought this was just a normal part of growing up but had no idea he was into drugs. He has said that he was stupid and it was the first time he has taken drugs but he hasn't told you why he took them or who he got them from.

Tom is a successful and popular boy. He is captain of his school football team and is desperate to join the Army. He intends to do this straight after school and has the selection next year. Now that he has recovered he is devastated by the thought that his medical history may stop him getting into the Army. One of your friends' sons was rejected last year because he suffers from asthma and you are well aware that they ask for a copy of the medical records.

For these reasons you want to ensure that this episode is deleted from his records. You really think that if he is given another chance he will realise how lucky he has been and not use drugs again. You don't think it can be right that one episode of stupidity should stop him joining the Army. If the doctor tells you that his records cannot be amended you will be very shocked – that is like a life sentence to him, taking away his dreams with one moment of ill judgement.

This is a difficult case examining a candidate's ability to empathise with Tom's mother and deal with a request that they may not know how to handle.

#### General manner

Polite, but fairly pushy – you really want your son to get a second chance.

# Relative scenario 9

## Candidate instructions

In this exercise, you will be consulted by a patient's relative in an acute hospital setting.

**Your task: you have a total of 10 minutes (including reading time) to complete this exercise. When you are ready to begin the consultation, please invite the relative to enter the room.**

You are an FY2 doctor working on an acute medical ward. Mrs Jones' son has asked to see you. Mrs Jones is ready for discharge following her admission last week with pneumonia, which required intravenous antibiotics. She is due to be discharged back to her nursing home.

## Actor instructions

Your 92-year-old mother is currently in hospital recovering from pneumonia. She seems so much brighter and happier now and has, in your mind, received excellent care in hospital. This has highlighted how terrible her nursing home is. She has been living in the nursing home since your father, her main carer, died 18 months ago. She has dementia and was not coping at home.

You feel that the nursing staff at the home do not care. Some of the things you have seen there have horrified you. You have witnessed residents being pushed back into their chairs and others manhandled across the room. You do realise that it is hard dealing with confused patients, but some nurses manage to do it in such a kind and caring way while others are frankly aggressive.

Prior to this admission you had spoken to your mother on a few occasions and noticed that she seemed breathless and had been coughing. You had asked the nurses what they were doing about it and they had dismissed you, saying that she was fine. Clearly, given how unwell she was on admission, they were mistaken.

You live in Manchester. You had to move there 1 year ago and feel so guilty to have left your mother behind. You work as a teacher and can only visit once every 2 to 3 weeks during term time. You have a wife and two children and know that your mother misses seeing the family.

Last year you talked to her GP and decided that it would be too unsettling to move your mother, but now you feel you can't let her go back to the nursing home. You have started to look for nursing homes near you in Manchester. You haven't made a final decision yet but you want her to stay in hospital until you find her a suitable home.

This case tests a candidate's ability to deal with potentially serious allegations of misconduct and a difficult request for the patient to stay in hospital until a new nursing home is found.

### General manner

Polite, but angry with yourself for letting your mother live in such a bad nursing home. A bit shocked and upset if informed that she can't stay in hospital.

# Relative scenario 10

## Candidate instructions

In this exercise, you will be consulted by a patient's relative in a GP setting.

**Your task: you have a total of 10 minutes (including reading time) to complete this exercise. When you are ready to begin the consultation, please invite the relative to enter the room.**

You are an FY2 doctor working in general practice. Hilary West, Ms West's daughter has booked an appointment to discuss her mother's care. Mrs West was visited by another GP at the practice a few weeks ago. The notes read:

> 94-year-old woman with severe bilateral knee osteoarthritis that makes it hard for her to climb stairs. She was previously seen by a knee surgeon who felt that she was too frail to benefit from surgery. Her daughter is her main carer. Plan: continue analgesia and organise social services assessment.

## Actor instructions

You are Hilary West, the 61-year-old daughter of Dorothy West. You need to see the doctor because you are really struggling to cope with looking after your mother. Your mother is very frail, age has taken its toll and she's becoming weaker each month. She suffers with severe pain in both knees and paracetamol, the only painkillers she seems able to tolerate, doesn't seem to be working.

You live in the same village and go over every morning to help her get washed and dressed and then in the evening you cook her dinner and help her to bed. Increasingly you have found this difficult and despite all of your attempts you just can't seem to get your mother to agree to have carers look after her. This is probably because your father had such a bad experience with carers when he was ill. The carers changed every day and came at ridiculous hours – one day they tried to put him to bed at 5 pm. They seemed to be in an enormous rush and he really hated it.

Things have come to a head now. You had an episode of postmenopausal bleeding and have been diagnosed with endometrial cancer. You haven't told your mother because you don't want to worry her, but you have been advised that you won't be able to do any manual work, lifting, etc. for at least 6 weeks after the hysterectomy, which is planned for next week. You know that your mother will refuse care and you will spend all of your recovery time worrying about her. In fact, you think that the stress of looking after your mother has probably caused your cancer.

You work as a librarian in the adjacent town. You have two brothers who live abroad, who you speak with often but they are, of course, not around to help.

This case is designed to see how a candidate explores the relative's issues and underlying concerns. It requires the formulation of sensitive solutions and an empathic approach.

### General manner

Exhausted and stressed. You will be relieved if the difficulties you are experiencing are acknowledged and sensible solutions discussed.

# Relative scenario 11

## Candidate instructions

In this exercise, you will be consulted by a patient's relative in a GP setting.

### Your task: you have a total of 10 minutes (including reading time) to complete this exercise. When you are ready to begin the consultation, please invite the relative to enter the room.

Mrs Jameson comes to see you regarding her husband who is a consultant anaesthetist at the local hospital.

## Actor instructions

You have asked to see the doctor to speak about your husband. You know that he would hate you to be talking about him, but you really don't know who you should ask for help. Over the past 6 months your husband has been sleeping poorly, is often irritable and has been drinking every night. You have tried to talk to him but he denies that there is a problem, despite it impacting on your home life. Your children have picked up on it, he seems constantly exhausted and you rarely have a sensible conversation now.

He has stopped meeting his friends, playing squash and going to the gym. These were things he previously loved to do. He drinks a bottle of wine and three or four whiskies at night and this seems to be increasing. You don't think he drinks during the day but suspect he stops off at the pub after work because he often smells of alcohol when he arrives home.

You really don't know why he has become like this or how you can help him. You are aware that he is under investigation at work after a patient died unexpectedly in the middle of a routine operation and he always complains about the lack of funding for the ITU department. However, he started to act strangely before any of this happened.

You really don't know what to do. You think he needs to see a doctor but how can you persuade him?

This case requires a candidate to empathise with a concerned relative, explore what is going on (including ensuring that there are no risks to patients if he continues to work) and trying to come up with ways of helping his wife persuade him to get help.

### General manner

Worried and concerned that your husband will be upset with you talking about this.

## Relative scenario 12

### Candidate instructions

In this exercise, you will be consulted by a patient's relative in a GP setting.

### Your task: you have a total of 10 minutes (including reading time) to complete this exercise. When you are ready to begin the consultation, please invite the relative to enter the room.

Paul's mother (Mrs Johnson) asks to see you. Paul is 8 years old and has been seen in the practice a few times over the past few years with upper respiratory tract infections.

### Actor instructions

You have come to ask the doctor for an epinephrine intramuscular injectable pen for your son. You think that it is safest if he has one. Paul's cousin was stung by a bee last week and was rushed to hospital with a severe allergic reaction. He is OK now, but has been given an injectable pen to carry with him at all times. You feel it is safest for Paul also to have one and so you have come to ask the doctor to prescribe this.

You are a 36-year-old woman. You only have one child. Paul's brother died when he was only 3 months old (due to cot death). You can't bear to think of anything happening to Paul and you try to protect him in any way possible. Your husband thinks you are overly cautious and doesn't think Paul needs a pen, but when your sister phoned to say that her son had been rushed to hospital and was really unwell it set off all of these fears and worries in you.

Paul has never really had any allergies and you think he probably has been stung by bees before, but you read that allergies can develop at any time.

You are expecting a bit of a battle with the doctor. You know the NHS is short of money and that the doctor won't want to prescribe an injectable pen, but you are willing to pay for it because cost shouldn't be an issue where your son's health is concerned. You are able to listen and accept any other reason for not prescribing the pen if you feel the doctor has understood your concerns and if the explanation seems adequate.

This case is more than just responding to a prescription request. It requires the candidate to explore and deal with the reasons behind maternal anxiety.

### General manner

Anxious and pushy.

# Relative scenario 13

## Candidate instructions

In this exercise, you will be consulted by a patient's relative in a GP setting.

**Your task: you have a total of 10 minutes (including reading time) to complete this exercise. When you are ready to begin the consultation, please invite the relative to enter the room.**

Mrs Josie Owens (36 years old) has booked in to see you to discuss her husband's recent consultation at your practice.

## Actor instructions

You have come to see the doctor to ask whether your husband has been treated for *Chlamydia*. You recently developed pelvic pain and vaginal discharge and went to a walk-in clinic. Swabs taken there showed *Chlamydia* infection.

You told your husband, who went and got tested and he has told you that his result was negative, so he has accused you of having an affair. You have not had an affair and last had sex with someone else 9 years ago before you met him. Initially, you were so keen to make your husband believe that you hadn't had an affair that you didn't even think that *he* might have been unfaithful. You now feel that he must have passed the infection to you and that he is lying about his negative test.

Your relationship has been strained for the past few years. Your husband has taken a high-pressured job as a corporate lawyer. He works late and often at weekends and so you hardly spend any quality time together.

You don't know what to do. You want to know for sure that his test was negative and are hoping the doctor can confirm this. You also want to know how else you could have contracted this infection. You aren't surprised if the doctor refuses to disclose your husband's medical records.

This is a difficult case designed to see how well a candidate can talk about relationship problems and help an obviously distressed lady.

### General manner

Upset.

## Relative scenario 14

### Candidate instructions

In this exercise, you will be consulted by a patient's relative in a GP setting.

**Your task: you have a total of 10 minutes (including reading time) to complete this exercise. When you are ready to begin the consultation, please invite the relative to enter the room.**

Mr Ward has booked in to see you to discuss his 15-year-old daughter, Isabelle. Isabelle was seen by a colleague at the surgery 3 months ago and prescribed the oral contraceptive pill.

### Actor instructions

You are Mr Jeremy Ward. You have come to see the doctor to discuss your daughter, Isabelle, who is 15 years old.

You found a packet of contraceptive pills in Isabelle's room yesterday and you are furious that they have been prescribed without your consent. You can't believe the doctor could condone underage sex and are shocked that you and your wife were not consulted.

You know Isabelle has a boyfriend but you are shocked that she would think about having sex at such a young age. Isabelle is away on a German exchange trip at the moment so you haven't been able to challenge her.

You have always had a good relationship with Isabelle, and you feel like you are a close, loving family. There have obviously been the usual arguments but nothing more than you would expect with a social, independent teenage daughter.

You are angry and cross, and you struggle to understand how a GP would prescribe your daughter the pill without consulting you. She is underage after all. If the GP stays calm and offers appropriate explanations you can calm down.

This is a case designed to test whether a candidate is familiar with legal issues surrounding management of teenagers in general practice. Candidates need to know about Fraser competence and confidentiality, and how to put this into practice.

### General manner

Hostile.

# Relative scenario 15

## Candidate instructions

In this exercise, you will be consulted by a patient's relative in a GP setting.

## Your task: you have a total of 10 minutes (including reading time) to complete this exercise. When you are ready to begin the consultation, please invite the relative to enter the room.

Mr Thomas Brett, 45 years old, has booked in to see you to discuss his wife's care. Mrs Brett has been seen in the practice recently and she was also discussed at an multidisciplinary team meeting you attended. She has metastatic breast cancer.

## Actor instructions.

You are Thomas Brett, a 45-year-old man. Your wife was diagnosed with breast cancer 18 months ago and she has become increasingly unwell over the past 4 months. Last week her oncologist told you that the cancer had spread into her bones and liver and that any treatment would be aimed at controlling the disease; a cure would not be possible.

You haven't told your children yet (who are aged 7 and 8 years old) although you know that they realise she is not well. You are trying to support your wife as much as possible. Your employers (a small building firm) have been very understanding and have told you to take as much time off as you need to, but you do worry that you are imposing on them and they won't survive without you.

You are not really sure why you have come to see the GP. You want to be strong for your family but you feel like you can't carry on like this. You believe you are being weak if you cry or get upset because you think you should just pick yourself up and carry on.

You really want to discuss how you should go about telling your children and whether there is any support available to them. You also want to know what will happen when your wife has radiotherapy and how it will make her feel.

Hopefully the doctor will reassure you that the way that you are feeling is normal, that you shouldn't feel like you have to cope alone and that you can accept help.

This case tests a candidate's ability to listen and approach a difficult and upsetting situation.

## General manner

Upset but feeling guilty for showing 'weakness'.

## Healthcare professional scenario 1

### Candidate instructions

In this exercise you will be consulted by a hospital colleague in an acute hospital setting.

**Your task: you have a total of 10 minutes (including reading time) to complete this exercise. When you are ready to begin the consultation, please invite your colleague to enter the room.**

You are an SHO in an emergency department. Sue Smith, one of the nursing staff, asks you to meet her before your shift is due to start.

### Actor instructions

You are Sue Smith. You have been a nurse in this emergency department for over 3 years. Recently you have felt that you are being singled out and bullied. One of the ward sisters, Jane, keeps telling you off in front of other colleagues and asks you to do unpleasant jobs, such as cleaning patients who have vomited or soiled themselves, much more often compared to other colleagues.

Yesterday the underground was delayed so you got to work 10 minutes late, and when you arrived she shouted at you in front of patients and staff and refused to listen to the reason for your lateness.

You think that her attitude toward you changed after you witnessed her giving the incorrect medication to a patient. You ensured an incident form was filled out and she seems to have taken objection to this. You didn't want to put blame on her as anyone could make such a mistake, but so that everybody could learn from these mistakes and avoid them happening in the future.

You have never had problems at work before and have enjoyed it thus far, but you are thinking of trying to move to a different department if things do not improve. It is affecting your performance as you are constantly nervous and you are getting upset about it at home. You live with two other flatmates who are your friends, but they are busy with their own work. Your family live nearby but you do not confide in them, as you never want to burden anyone. You used to go out socially with colleagues, but do so less frequently since this started and therefore you spend more time alone at home.

The last time you experienced anything like this was when you were bullied at school. You feel the same now – that it is somehow your fault. Everything was fine when you changed schools and you are sure it will be fine if you move departments.

You do not know what to do and want advice from another colleague who isn't a nurse because you are worried it will get back to Jane. You are concerned that if you make a complaint, things will only get worse and you'll get a bad reference.

This case is designed for the candidate to show support and kindness towards a distressed colleague.

**General manner**

Wronged, fed-up, upset.

# Healthcare professional scenario 2

## Candidate instructions

In this exercise you will be consulted by a hospital colleague in a hospital setting.

**Your task: you have a total of 10 minutes (including reading time) to complete this exercise. When you are ready to begin the consultation, please invite your colleague to enter the room.**

You are an oncology SHO. Lizzie, a physiotherapist on the ward, has asked to meet you during the 10-minute break in the weekly multidisciplinary team meeting for a private chat about an oncology patient, Mr Franks, who died this morning.

## Actor instructions

You are Lizzie. You have recently started working as a physiotherapist in the oncology and palliative care department. One of your patients (Mr Franks) died this morning. He was a palliative patient with end-stage metastatic lung cancer and you have found this event terribly upsetting.

You had been giving him regular chest physiotherapy to keep him more comfortable but throughout his stay he was breathless and often seemed to be in pain. You feel very upset as he was a lovely man, only 58 years old, and you had got to know him and his family quite well. You feel very emotional and are worried that this could affect your work. You are also worried about how you will cope with the deaths of other patients. Everybody else seems able to cope, and are hardly affected by these things, but you ended up crying for over an hour when you found out he had died.

Your mother died of pancreatic cancer 5 years ago and you remember her being in a great deal of pain. This job seems to be bringing back memories of her death. You live with your boyfriend who is a busy lawyer, so you try not to bring up work at home. Your father lives nearby but hasn't mentioned your mother's death for 3 years and you don't feel able to talk to him about it.

You have not told any of your physiotherapist colleagues because you are worried they will think you are being oversensitive.

This case tests a candidate's ability to deal with an upset, worried colleague. It requires empathy and reassurance and for the candidate to explore the underlying reasons for her distress.

### General manner

Shocked, upset and wondering whether you can cope in this job.

## Healthcare professional scenario 3

### Candidate instructions
In this exercise, you will be consulted by a GP colleague in a surgery.

**Your task: you have a total of 10 minutes (including reading time) to complete this exercise. When you are ready to begin the consultation, please invite your colleague to enter the room.**

You are a salaried GP at a practice in West London. Karen Holt, one of the receptionists, would like to speak to you after work today about Dr Dias, the GP registrar. She only has 10 minutes to spare as she needs to pick up her children from school.

### Actor instructions
You are Karen Holt, an experienced GP receptionist who has worked at the same practice for 4 years. You have noticed that Dr Dias, the new GP registrar who started 2 months ago, has been behaving a bit strangely. Over the past 4 weeks he has been coming to work late at least 3 times a week and has been rude to a few patients who have subsequently complained to you. You have had to apologise on his behalf several times.

Dr Dias has also snapped at many of the reception staff, including you, and has not been doing his share of repeat prescriptions on time, causing delays for patients. He is taking a long time to see each patient, his appointments run extremely late and on a few occasions has come to work looking extremely unkempt.

His trainer has been on holiday for 2 weeks. You have asked Dr Dias if everything is OK on a few occasions but he reassured you that everything is fine. You are very worried about him and how his behaviour may be affecting patient care. Other people have talked to you about him but have not done anything about the situation.

You really think one of the doctors should have noticed and should be sorting things out already because it is not fair on the staff or the patients.

This case examines a candidate's ability to come up with a solution for dealing with an underperforming colleague, ensuring that patient care is not at risk.

#### General manner
Concerned, worried about the effect the registrar's behaviour is having on patients and staff.

# Healthcare professional scenario 4

## Candidate instructions
In this exercise you will be consulted by a colleague in a hospital setting.

**Your task: you have a total of 10 minutes (including reading time) to complete this exercise. When you are ready to begin the consultation, please invite your colleague to enter the room.**

You are an FY2 working in an emergency department. One of the healthcare assistants would like to speak to you today during your 10-minute coffee break.

## Actor instructions
You are Kate Cleveland, a healthcare assistant in the emergency department. You have overheard another doctor making racist comments about patients they have seen in the department. Examples of the comments include: 'I wish they would go back to their own country' and 'How come they can't learn English?'.

You were very shocked and upset by this and want to speak to someone about it. You haven't told anyone else because you are worried that people will not believe you. You were initially just going to ignore it because you don't want to cause trouble and fear you could lose your job or be treated badly.

Last year one of the nurses reported that another nurse had given the wrong fluids to a patient and she ended up feeling forced to leave because no one seemed to trust her after that. You are a single mother and couldn't possibly afford to lose this job. Things are hard enough as it is and your daughter is settled into the hospital crèche now.

Ideally you do not want anyone to know you have raised this concern but you do want it to go further. You are hoping that the doctor can inform someone on your behalf.

This case tests a candidate's ability to reassure a colleague that racism is completely unacceptable, that she is right to raise the issue and to come up with a feasible plan.

### General manner
Quiet, visibly upset and shocked when you recall what you have heard.

# Healthcare professional scenario 5

## Candidate instructions

In this exercise you will be consulted by a colleague in a hospital setting.

**Your task: you have a total of 10 minutes (including reading time) to complete this exercise. When you are ready to begin the consultation, please invite your colleague to enter the room.**

You are an orthopaedic FY2. A senior nurse, Bill Tibbs, asked to speak to you yesterday but you were called off to an emergency so you agreed to meet with him today.

## Actor instructions

You are Bill, a senior nurse, who has been working at this hospital for 15 years. You are very experienced in dealing with postoperative patients and have become increasingly worried about Mr Blackbridge, a consultant surgeon who started at the trust 6 months ago.

You have noticed that the complication rate, particularly of wound infections, in his patients is very high. You also are very concerned about his attitude towards some of the nursing staff and junior doctors. He has not shouted at you or been particularly rude but he but has ignored your concerns on a number of occasions and he always leaves it to his junior doctors to review his postoperative cases. In fact, he hardly ever sees his own patients and you are sure that some of them have never even met him.

You know you have a duty to report your concerns but don't really like the idea of being a 'whistleblower' because you are worried how other doctors and staff will react towards you.

Ideally, you would like the FY2 to speak to the team and to raise the issue with Mr Blackbridge but you are also open to other suggestions.

This case tests a candidate's ability to gather all of the information and then come up with a sensible solution to a delicate problem.

### General manner

Confident senior nurse. You feel you owe it to your patients to stand up for them and are a bit annoyed with yourself for not mentioning it earlier.

# Healthcare professional scenario 6

## Candidate instructions

In this exercise you will be consulted by a hospital colleague in a hospital setting.

**Your task: you have a total of 10 minutes (including reading time) to complete this exercise. When you are ready to begin the consultation, please invite your colleague to enter the room.**

You are a medical registrar. One of the nurses has some concerns regarding the medical consultant, Dr Thomas. She has not disclosed any other information but said she needed to speak to you urgently. You have 10 minutes before handover in which to speak to her.

## Actor instructions

You are Jenny, a senior sister on the ward. You were going to use the printer in the doctors' office on the ward last week and caught the consultant, Dr Thomas, kissing his FY2, Stephanie. They were very embarrassed and apologised to you, and Dr Thomas has since approached you to request that you are discrete about the situation.

You think he is married with children and whilst you think it is wrong that he is having an affair, you know that it is not your business. You are most concerned because you have noticed that he has been treating Stephanie very differently to other junior doctors and you now understand why. He has been her supervisor and has been filling out all her assessment forms for her, which you feel is unprofessional.

You do not know how to proceed and always have got on well with this consultant, who you respect as a very good doctor. You have no concerns about his patient care, which you feel is excellent. You do not want to cause any problems but do not feel this is ethically appropriate and want some advice about how to proceed. You have had some sleepless nights worrying about what to do. You have spoken to your partner who thinks you should ignore it, but you feel it is too important to ignore. You are aware that if this is raised as an issue it will be obvious that it is you who reported it.

Candidates often find this case difficult and are surprised when the issue is first raised. A good candidate will appreciate the issues and explore them with the nurse before coming up with a reasonable solution.

## General manner

You are embarrassed to have raised the issue. You would like support, advice and reassurance.

# Healthcare professional scenario 7

## Candidate instructions

In this exercise you will be consulted by a colleague in a hospital setting.

**Your task: you have a total of 10 minutes (including reading time) to complete this exercise. When you are ready to begin the consultation, please invite your colleague to enter the room.**

You are a surgical FY2 doctor. You bumped into Caroline, a laboratory technician, when you dropped blood samples off at the pathology lab yesterday. She asked to speak to you and, as you were busy at the time, you agreed to meet her today.

## Actor instructions

You are Caroline, a laboratory technician, who has worked in the department for 5 years. Recently you have noticed an increase in inadequately labelled blood samples. You have kept an eye on things for the past month and have noticed that the majority of the errors are coming from the surgical wards.

You have to reject samples when they are not labelled correctly (they need a minimum of two identifiers e.g. name and DOB). You hate doing this because you know it puts more stress on the doctors and phlebotomists and it means that patient care can be affected.

On a few occasions, doctors have shouted at you when you have informed them that the samples could not be processed. You have started to dread going into work because of these problems and your partner at home has picked up on this and has urged you to do something about it.

You are not quite sure what to do but would appreciate any suggestions from the doctor. You want to be taken seriously and to have some solutions offered. You would be happy to help to complete an audit and would appreciate the doctor offering to hold a meeting, put posters up, etc., to highlight the need for adequate labelling of blood samples.

You feel upset when doctors shout at you – you are trying to do your job and are only following protocol to protect patient safety. It's not that hard to label a bottle correctly, is it?

This case is about recognising a problem and thinking of ways to manage it.

## General manner

Generally calm.

# Healthcare professional scenario 8

## Candidate instructions

In this exercise you will be consulted by a colleague in a hospital setting.

## Your task: you have a total of 10 minutes (including reading time) to complete this exercise. When you are ready to begin the consultation, please invite your colleague to enter the room.

You are an FY2 working on a surgical ward. The ward sister asks to see you urgently at the end of the ward round to discuss concerns she has about one of the FY1 doctors, Dr Peters. You haven't worked with Dr Peters yourself.

## Actor instructions

You are Fiona Walsh, ward sister on the surgical ward. You ask to see the doctor because you have concerns about the FY1, Dr Peters. You were on call with him this weekend and feel that he couldn't cope and probably wasn't competent enough to be doing the role.

He was asked to see a patient with a reduced urine output on Saturday and didn't do anything – he just kept asking you how much fluid you felt the patient should have. You had to point out that the patient was postoperative (bowel resection) and should probably have a blood sample taken. He also couldn't get blood out of two patients and left one patient with severely bruised arms after attempting a cannula insertion.

You really don't mind being asked for help, in fact you appreciate it when doctors recognise your experience, but in this case you feel that he really isn't ready for the role. You could accept it if he had just started as a doctor but he has been on the ward for 6 months now and you struggle to understand how he got this far.

You can't think of a case where a patient has come to serious harm as a result of his actions – other doctors always seem to come and help him out. You are, however, very worried that he is putting patients at risk and you feel he shouldn't be allowed to do on calls alone in future.

You know that this issue needs to be raised and you want to discuss it with someone else to see if they have ideas about how to approach it. You are amazed that no one else has realised that he isn't coping and acted upon this sooner.

This case tests a candidate's ability to deal with an underperforming colleague. They may not know the correct approach, but should establish the facts and have thoughts on what may be the most appropriate next step.

### General manner

Calm but concerned. You want something done and don't want your concerns to be ignored.

## Healthcare professional scenario 9

### Candidate instructions

In this exercise you will be consulted by a colleague in a hospital setting.

**Your task: you have a total of 10 minutes (including reading time) to complete this exercise. When you are ready to begin the consultation, please invite your colleague to enter the room.**

You are an FY2 doctor working on a medical ward. Julie, one of the staff nurses on the ward, asked to speak to you about a personal matter this morning. As you were busy at that time you agreed to meet her later in the day.

### Actor instructions

You are a 30-year-old staff nurse called Julie. You have asked to speak to one of the doctors because your father is unwell and you were hoping to get some advice. Three weeks ago your father was diagnosed with bowel cancer. He has had surgery and has been advised to have chemotherapy (although no metastases have been seen on imaging). You are extremely worried about him; he looks so unwell but keeps saying that he is doing fine.

Since his diagnosis you haven't really been sleeping. You are trying to stay strong for everyone. All of the family keep asking your advice because you are the only medically trained person around. Your parents live 10 miles away and you have been visiting them daily because your mother really isn't coping – she has chronic anxiety disorder and is constantly fearing the worst and overreacting to every small symptom your father develops. You are already extremely busy as a single parent to your 6-year-old daughter. You have an older brother but he lives in France and, whilst he is very supportive, he can't help a great deal.

You feel exhausted and hate seeing patients dying. You can't help but wonder whether you will be in their position, visiting your dying father in a few months' time. You are not really sure what to do and have tried not to take time off work – last year you had a month off with back pain and feel that it would be frowned upon and might affect your career if you had any more absences.

You would like to know how your father will be affected by the chemotherapy. You have never worked on an oncology ward before and don't have much experience of this. You would also appreciate discussing ways of coping and would welcome any suggestions about time off, etc.

This case examines a candidate's ability to counsel colleagues. It is important to be empathetic, supportive and suggest a few solutions but also to encourage the colleague to seek professional help from her own GP.

### General manner

Upset, tearful at times, thankful for appropriate advice.

# Healthcare professional scenario 10

## Candidate instructions
In this exercise you will be consulted by a colleague in a hospital setting.

## Your task: you have a total of 10 minutes (including reading time) to complete this exercise. When you are ready to begin the consultation, please invite your colleague to enter the room.
You are the mess president at your hospital. You bumped into Kim, one of the cleaners, in the mess while you were making coffee. She asked to speak to you and, as you were busy at the time, you agreed to meet her today.

## Actor instructions
You are Kim and you have been working in this hospital as a cleaner for the last 10 years. You are very frustrated by the state of the doctors' mess, which you feel is unacceptable. You have noticed doctors eating and not throwing their rubbish away, there are empty coffee cups all over the floor and unwashed mugs and plates left all over the room. You have to pick up patient lists (containing confidential information) and dispose of these correctly.

You spend 3 hours cleaning it each day whereas previously it had taken you 1 hour. Your manager is upset that you spend less time on the other areas of the hospital allocated to you. You have tried explaining the situation but he will not listen. You are very worried you will lose your job, so you have stayed beyond your time in order to finish your workload. As your husband has recently been made redundant, you are now the only breadwinner for the family.

Last week you put a polite notice up in the mess asking people to clean up after themselves. You are extremely upset as someone wrote 'Do it yourself – that's your job' on it.

You have asked to speak to the mess president about this as you have had enough.

This case tests a candidate's ability to communicate effectively with the cleaner, understand her concerns and reassure her that something can and must be done.

### General manner
Initially angry. Doesn't give too much information away early on but will explain concerns if the doctor acknowledges the problems and seems supportive and empathetic.

# Healthcare professional scenario 11

## Candidate instructions

In this exercise you will be consulted by a colleague in a hospital setting.

**Your task: you have a total of 10 minutes (including reading time) to complete this exercise. When you are ready to begin the consultation, please invite your colleague to enter the room.**

You are an FY2 doctor working on a medical ward. Mr Paul Yates, infection control nurse, has asked to see you to discuss a few infection control issues.

## Actor instructions

You are Paul Yates, a 47-year-old infection control nurse in the hospital. You have asked to see the doctor because you have noticed a lot of the doctors on the wards are not obeying hand infection control rules. Most of the junior doctors still wear watches, hardly any roll up their sleeves and not all doctors wash their hands between patients. You find this so frustrating. Surely protecting patients from germs that doctors carry should be a priority. Do they not realise they are causing harm? You have spoken to a few doctors and told them to remove watches, roll sleeves up, etc. but they have acted as if it is a big joke – some of them seemed to pull faces behind your back.

You have also noticed, although you know it is not really your business, that some of the junior doctors seem very casual. A few of the female doctors are wearing very low cut tops and short skirts. What happened to professionalism?

You find your job very stressful; there was been an MRSA outbreak recently and on the back of the *Clostridium difficile* outbreak that closed two wards last year, the hospital managers are pressuring you. You really feel that unless things improve you will get sacked but you don't really think there is much more you can do; all the policies and procedures are in place but members of staff are not following them.

You really want advice as to what can be done to help people conform. You are on the verge of adopting a 'name and shame policy'. Ideally you would like a sensible discussion about what can be done, good suggestions to be made and the doctors to understand how stressful it is for you.

This case tests a candidate's ability to demonstrate empathy, build rapport with the infection control nurse and come up with workable solutions to the problem.

### General manner

Frustrated, don't know what else to do, stressed; would be calmed and thankful if the doctor addresses concerns.

# Healthcare professional scenario 12

## Candidate instructions

In this exercise you will be consulted by a colleague in a GP setting.

## Your task: you have a total of 10 minutes (including reading time) to complete this exercise. When you are ready to begin the consultation, please invite your colleague to enter the room.

You are an FY2 doctor working in general practice. Sophie Lesley, practice nurse, has asked to see you briefly after the morning surgery.

## Actor instructions

You are Sophie Lesley, a 35-year-old practice nurse. You have asked to see the doctor because you are 7 weeks pregnant and suffering with quite severe morning sickness, and as a result you are struggling to cope with your surgeries.

You have been trying to get pregnant for 3 years and last year had a miscarriage at 10 weeks gestation. You know it is stupid but you felt such a failure. All of your friends have children and your husband, who is very supportive, is desperate to be a father. You were thrilled when you found out that you were pregnant again but now you feel so anxious that something may go wrong.

You don't want anyone to know that you are pregnant in case you have another miscarriage, but you have been sick in between patients and have to work at a slower pace. Last week one of the partners told you off for not completing all of your administrative work. At the moment you can hardly manage to see your patients, let alone keep up with all of the paperwork. Over the last few days getting into work on time has been hard because you keep being sick in the mornings.

Your husband works as an electrician but things aren't really going so well with his work so your income is very important.

You hope the doctor has some suggestions and are very keen for him to agree that the conversation should be confidential.

This case tests the ability of a candidate to engage with the nurse, in order for her to open up. Good listening skills and empathy are important attributes to demonstrate.

### General manner

Tired, anxious, looking for reassurance and help.

# Healthcare professional scenario 13

## Candidate instructions
In this exercise you will be consulted by a colleague in a GP setting.

## Your task: you have a total of 10 minutes (including reading time) to complete this exercise. When you are ready to begin the consultation, please invite your colleague to enter the room.

Sue, head receptionist at the practice where you are working as an FY2, has asked to see you.

## Actor instructions
You are Sue, a 37-year-old head receptionist at the practice. You wanted to speak to the doctor to get advice. Last week you saw the new health visitor take £10 out of the petty cash box when she was putting her temporary car permit back (they are stored in the same place). You did think about ignoring it but it has really been bugging you and you don't feel you can trust her anymore.

You haven't told Keith, the practice manager. You had a big falling out with him a few months ago, when he wrongly accused you of messing up the appointment system and of being rude to patients. This ended up being discussed in a partnership meeting. In the end the partners thought the practice manager was in the wrong and supported you. You haven't mentioned this recent incident to the partners yet because you don't necessarily want it to go any further. It is stressful enough having a practice manager hating you, let alone the health visitors too.

You aren't really enjoying work at the moment – the difficult working relationship with Keith is taking its toll. You don't have a partner and usually really love work. You love the fact you were previously so well-regarded and felt an essential part of the practice, but things do seem to have changed.

Overall you want to talk through the options and get some support. You don't want to cause trouble but don't know how it can be ignored.

This case is testing how a candidate responds to a situation of potential theft in a professional manner. It requires good listening and problem solving skills, as well as demonstrating empathy towards the receptionist, who is also having problems with another member of staff.

### General manner
Quiet, pragmatic, appreciating time to talk.

# Healthcare professional scenario 14

## Candidate instructions

In this exercise you will be consulted by a colleague in a hospital setting.

**Your task: you have a total of 10 minutes (including reading time) to complete this exercise. When you are ready to begin the consultation, please invite your colleague to enter the room.**

Rebecca Coley, a physiotherapist on your ward, asks to see you (a respiratory FY2 doctor) after work.

## Actor instructions

You are Rebecca, a 28-year-old physiotherapist on the respiratory ward. You have asked to speak to the doctor because you are really upset. You have just attended a lunchtime meeting where everybody was informed that disciplinary procedures would be taken against anyone making comments about the hospital, staff or patients on social networking sites.

Managers said that they had already been informed of a few examples and would be following these up. This has come as a total shock to you – you have never thought about it before and know you have made some pretty derogatory comments on one such website. As soon as the meeting ended you deleted the posts but you are worried that you they will already have been seen by the managers.

Most of your comments are based around how terrible the nurses are. You really feel for the patients who are too sick to feed themselves, when nurses sit around the nurses' station gossiping all of the time. They never offer to help, you always have to ask, and, bar a few exceptions, help is only provided reluctantly. You know it is not right but you have made impulsive comments on one social networking site.

You have not only experienced bad nursing care at work, but also personally when your mother was admitted to hospital. She was left in pain for hours, with the nurses simply sitting around the nurses' station.

You are now so upset – what if your comments have been seen? What should you do?

This case requires the candidate to be open, reassuring and able to calm the physiotherapist down. It also requires the candidate to behave in a professional manner regarding the use of social networking sites for work-related discussion and how to solve this problem in a sensible way.

### General manner

Upset, confused and anxious.

# Healthcare professional scenario 15

## Candidate instructions

In this exercise you will be consulted by a colleague in a hospital setting.

**Your task: you have a total of 10 minutes (including reading time) to complete this exercise. When you are ready to begin the consultation, please invite your colleague to enter the room.**

You are an FY2 doctor working on a medical ward. Mrs Marilyn Jones, the ward clerk on your ward has asked to have a private word with you regarding your FY2 colleague, Dr Hemley.

## Actor instructions

You are Marilyn Jones, a 56-year-old ward clerk, who has worked on the medical ward (health care of the elderly) for the past 12 years. You really enjoy your job but are having problems with one of the FY2s and, after much thought, you have decided to raise your concerns.

Dr Hemley has been off work for the past week. He calls you each morning to say that he is still feeling unwell and you have just taken another such call from him. Last night you saw him at the cinema having fun with friends and he had obviously been drinking. When he called this morning you were about to mention this to him but decided against it.

You have had a few problems with him in the past. He seems to think he is better than anyone else; he doesn't seem to want to work on the ward and takes objection to any request for him to do anything. On a few occasions he has shouted at you and you now fear bleeping him because of the response you might get.

You don't think anyone else has realised because on ward rounds he always comes across as enthusiastic and caring. You don't think he should be allowed to get away with it. He shouldn't be calling in sick if he is not – you know it is putting a massive strain on the other doctors and it doesn't seem fair.

You don't want him to realise that you have made the complaint and ideally would prefer someone else to report it on your behalf.

This case requires a good candidate to be open and non-judgemental when discussing the concerns of the ward clerk about another colleague. It is important to make her feel that her concern is being taken seriously and to come up with sensible solutions to the problem.

### General manner

Infuriated.

# Chapter 5

# Transcribed consultations

This chapter presents a transcription of a well-performed consultation for each of the exercises described in Chapter 4. Where specific skills have been demonstrated by the candidate, these are flagged on the right-hand side of the page. Use these as a resource for exploring ways of approaching specific situations and as a source of succinct phrases to employ in your own consultations.

## Patient scenario 1

| Transcript | Skills demonstrated |
| --- | --- |
| **D:** Good morning Mr Ward, come on in. | Used patient's name |
| **P:** Thank you. | |
| **D:** One of the nurses has said you wanted to speak to me – how can I help? | Open question |
| **P:** I've just been discharged after the ward rounds and I don't know if you were on it but I'm still worried about it. | |
| **D:** OK then, could just tell me a bit more about what you're worried about? | Open question |
| **P:** Well I've been given the inhalers, I've been told everything will get better. Well, it won't get better but will improve and I'm just unsure about everything because I still get out of breath. | |
| **D:** That's fine, if you could just go right back to the situation before you came into the hospital and what's been going on since then? | Exploring context |
| **P:** I'm quite wheezy, well my wife has been saying I'm wheezy, and I saw my GP when I had this chesty cough. He put this thing on my finger and listened to my chest and said I had to go into hospital. And I got admitted; good job really. They gave me the antibiotics, and did some tests. But they said it's because of my smoking. | |

**D:** So what did they say that you had?

Establishing prior knowledge

**P:** They said I got something like asthma, but because of smoking.

**D:** And what do you understand by that?

Checking understanding

**P:** Well it just means that I'm a bit puffy.

**D:** Do you want me to go through that in more detail because it sounds as though it might be a lot to understand?

Signposting

**P:** Yes, OK.

**D:** It sounds like you have been breathless and wheezy for a while, but things got worse before you were admitted. This is probably because an infection made an existing, underlying condition called 'COPD' worse. Has anyone mentioned this to you before?

**P:** No, no.

**D:** Well it sounds like the infection has been treated because you're not coughing as much and you don't seem unwell anymore. But we think you have an underlying condition that affects your lungs and affects smokers which may be why you have developed this. It makes it more difficult for you to breathe than other people with healthier lungs. This is why we have started you on this medication, the inhalers.

Explaining without jargon

**P:** OK.

**D:** How bad do you think things were before you came in when you were at home?

**P:** Well they were quite bad, but I just thought it was a chest infection. I was told it can't be cured.

**D:** Tell me a bit more about your smoking, is that something you do at the moment?

Closed question exploring related issue

**P:** Oh yes, I've always been smoking, probably smoke too much. I tried to quit but that didn't work.

**D:** How do you feel now about giving up smoking now that you've had this diagnosis?

**P:** I should give up, but it's easier said than done.

**D:** Absolutely. It's really about finding the right time, when you're ready to stop and you can always go to your GP when you're ready. There are always things they can help you with. Is there anything that you're particularly worried about? You seem quite anxious.

Empathy
Exploring ICE
Picking up emotional/non-verbal cue

**P:** Yes I'm worried that things would just get worse, you think of the big C, cancer. My dad had cancer and also I just don't always want to be breathless.

**D:** COPD may get worse if you carry on smoking, so that's something you should address at some point. I'm sorry to hear about your father's cancer. Is that something that's been playing on your mind?

Showing sensitivity and empathy

**P:** Yes it has to be honest, I know I shouldn't smoke, this has just hit me, and I've never been in hospital before. Now I've got this lung problem; what's stopping me getting cancer?

**D:** I can understand why you are worrying about this especially if you have a history of cancer in the family, and the smoking. But I can assure you that the tests that have been done today haven't actually shown that you have cancer. Where cancer is associated with smoking and COPD they are two completely different diseases. So I hope I can reassure you that it's not something you have at the moment. Does that make you feel a little more at ease?

Empathy

Explaining results

Reflecting back (concerns of cancer)

**P:** Yes a little bit better, well that's good. Because no one said I didn't have cancer before.

**D:** Oh I understand. You were also saying about how you were a little worried about how this is going to progress at home. Do you want to tell me a little more about that?

Reflecting back on an earlier concern and picking up on cues

**P:** Well, it's been difficult because my daughter has been staying at home, while I've been at the hospital looking after my wife. And she can't carry on doing that, she has a family of her own. I've been struggling with it to be honest. I'm just worried about what's going to happen if anything happens to me.

**D:** Do you mind if I ask about your wife, how is she?

**P:** She's got diabetes and she has not been well at the moment. She has this big ulcer on her foot that the district nurse has been coming to sort out. She's quite immobile with that really. I have to give her a hand with most things.

**D:** You mention that your daughter has been helping out while you have been here – does she usually help out?

**P:** She does a bit but I usually manage most things.

**D:** How are you coping at home?

**P:** Yes I'm managing at the moment, with the breathing problems it was quite hard but I managed.

**D:** Other than your daughter and the district nurses, do you have any other help?

**P:** No.

**D:** Well we can see if we can get you more help. I could organise for you and your wife to be seen by a social worker to see if we can organise a carer to come in. Would you find this helpful?

**P:** OK – that would be brilliant.

**D:** Now you're on the inhalers how are you feeling in yourself?

**P:** Yes, I'm good. Ready to go home now, I think I was just a bit worried about everything.

**D:** Do you feel that your breathing is better controlled?

**P:** Yes, still get a bit out of breath but it is much better now.

**D:** Do you feel happy with how to use your medications?

**P:** Yeah the specialist nurse came round and showed me everything.

Establishing social situation and impact of illness.

Problem solving and involving patient in decisions

| | |
|---|---|
| **D:** If you do have any issues in the future you can go to your GP and I think it will be good if we arrange a follow up in the clinic here in a few weeks time, just to make sure you are OK with everything. I will get someone to come round and have a chat with you about maybe having a carer. How does that sound? | Checking understanding<br>Organising follow-up |
| **P:** Yeah, that all sounds good. Thanks. | |

## Patient scenario 2

| Transcript | Skills demonstrated |
|---|---|
| **D:** Hello Mr Xavi, do come in, how may I help? | Used patient's name |
| **P:** I have a letter from the surgery to come in and talk about my results because they're abnormal. | |
| **D:** OK, well why don't you take me through what has been going on? | Establishing patient's understanding with open question |
| **P:** Oh God, are they really bad? | |
| **D:** No, I think it will be good if I can get the full picture of what's been going on and we can put these results into context. | |
| **P:** Well I came in last week with chest pain and I had to go into hospital and they did all these tests, they said I was fine but I thought I was having a heart attack. | |
| **D:** That must have been very stressful for you. | Picking up non verbal cue |
| **P:** Now I got this letter and it says something is abnormal. | |
| **D:** OK, so you've come in because you're concerned about this letter. Would you like me to go through the results now? | Reflecting back and signposting |
| **P:** Yes, please tell me exactly what's going on. | |
| **D:** Essentially we have asked you in to talk to you about your cholesterol results. Do you know anything about cholesterol? | Establishing prior knowledge |
| **P:** I know that if you have too much you can have a heart attack. | |

**D:** I can see that heart attacks are something you are worried about. Before we talk about this would you like me to explain a bit more about cholesterol to you?

Signposting

**P:** Yes please.

**D:** Cholesterol is really a type of fat in the blood, everyone has it. If you have higher levels than you should do, there's a slightly higher chance you will have a heart attack or stroke many years down the line. By no means is that inevitable. Cholesterol is what we call a risk factor, which we would like to control. It certainly doesn't mean that you will have a heart attack.

Explanation without jargon

**P:** Oh my, OK. Is it basically saying that I am fat?

**D:** Not at all. Cholesterol can be high for a few reasons. It can be high due to diet or it can be because it is just the way you are built in comparison to someone else.

**P:** Hmm, OK. So how bad is my cholesterol?

**D:** Well, your cholesterol level is a little high. Normally we aim for people to have it below 5, yours is at 7.2

**P:** Oh my God!

**D:** I don't want you to be overly anxious about this. We need to work out what is causing it and try to manage it. Would you mind if we go back and talk through what happened when you had the chest pain?

Reassurance and trying to understand patient's anxiety

**P:** Yes, so I was at home and was just watching TV a few weeks ago and I just got this chest pain. You know I've seen all the adverts that if you have chest pain you have to call an ambulance. They took me in and took all these tests that were all normal. They said that I may have had a panic attack but I didn't think I was at the time and they sent me home.

**D:** Yes, I've received all of the information from the hospital and that's all correct. They did a trace of your heart. You also went on the treadmill during your exercise test, which was also normal. Your blood pressure is also fine. So really we should look at this as a positive that we have picked up on your cholesterol. That chest pain was not a heart attack at all, but we can use this as an opportunity to talk about reducing the risk for the future. I noticed earlier that you seem anxious about heart attacks?

Reassurance

Picking up on emotional cue

P: I am anxious about it, you know I'm not young anymore and I live on my own. My neighbour died a few months ago of a sudden heart attack and she was younger than me. We were quite close and it has been on my mind.

D: Yes, I can see why that would be quite distressing for you. I hope that I have been able to reassure you. Really what we should be thinking about now is how to reduce the risk. Would you mind if we talk about your diet?

Signposting and health promotion

P: Yes that's fine.

D: How do you think your diet is?

P: Well it varies from day to day. I used to cook for my family, proper meals every day. But now I don't have a lot of money and I do tend to just get a burger on my way home from work or sometimes I just have beans on toast because I'm too tired to cook.

D: Do you drink alcohol?

P: I have a few glasses of wine a night, a bit more than I used to.

D: Do you smoke?

P: No, I've never smoked.

D: OK, well a few things come to mind. As I mentioned earlier cholesterol can be raised due to diet and alcohol. I think if you reduce your alcohol and improve your diet it will come down.

P: What sorts of food have high cholesterol?

D: Yes, that's a good question. Foods that contain a lot of cholesterol are red meats, dairy products, and certain shellfish. Red meat should only be had once a week ideally. Alcohol is also a major culprit. Maybe if you cut that down it will help. I can give you an information leaflet as to what to avoid?

Verbal and written information

P: Yeah that will be great.

D: OK just to summarise, you had this chest pain a few weeks ago which you went to hospital for. The tests they did all came back normal. The tests we did here for you showed raised cholesterol which is a little bit high. We discussed how that is a risk factor, so it doesn't mean you will have a heart attack, it just means we need to keep an eye on it. Do you have any family members nearby? | Summarising

P: Yes, well my son has just recently moved to Australia and I'm newly divorced. |

D: Sorry to hear that. How are you coping? | Empathy

P: It's OK, I'm managing. I don't have a lot of money since the divorce; I'm a cleaner so it's not regular work. That's why I'm worried if I collapsed at home no one would even notice. |

D: Well, I understand why you have been so worried about this but I hope I have reassured you that your cholesterol does not mean that you will have a heart attack. I think it will be good to check your cholesterol and blood pressure in a few months time. | Empathy and reassurance

P: OK, I'll book in to see you then. |

D: If there's anything else that you would like to discuss then don't hesitate to come in sooner. |

## Patient scenario 3

| Transcript | Skills demonstrated |
|---|---|
| D: Hello Miss Yetton, how can I help today? | Used patient's name |
| P: I don't know if you've seen my notes, I've seen a few doctors here. It's just really about my headaches. They are still there and I've tried everything I've been told to do. I really just need them to be sorted out once and for all. | |
| D: Tell me a bit more about these headaches. | Open question |
| P: It's just every day I have these horrible headaches, it gets worse and worse throughout the day and I feel like I have to go to sleep. That's the only time I feel like they go away. This has been going on for about 6 months. Always the same sort of thing, always really horrible round my head. The doctors here have told me to take all these different painkillers but nothing helps. | |

D: Yes I've got your notes and I see that you have had a few tests done ...

*Exploring understanding of tests*

P: Yes I was really worried. I was almost in tears one day. I've had this CT scan and they said everything was fine which I couldn't believe, but I still feel that I would be much happier if I could have an MRI. I've done a lot of reading and I know they are more sensitive and that they are better tests, and may be if I could see a neurologist. They may be able to help me with my headaches.

D: You mentioned you are worried and that you would feel comfortable with an MRI, what have you read that has led you to this decision?

*Exploring ideas*

P: Well, with the reading that I've done they say that the CT doesn't cover every region of the brain and small cancers can be missed. I'm just worried that I have a brain tumour and to me it seems like there has to be something serious because these headaches are unbearable.

D: Just to recap, you've had these headaches for 6 months that feel like a constant pressure. You have had a CT that didn't show any abnormalities. You would like to have an MRI just to confirm there is nothing wrong and there isn't a tumour. Does that all sound right?

*Summarising and checking patient's expectations*

P: Yes, I really would like the MRI.

D: We really need to think about what's going to help you the most. These headaches are ongoing and they are quite painful. I can understand why you are worried about a brain tumour. I suppose this would be a good time for me to reassure you as I don't think this is due to a brain tumour. Would you like me to explain why I think this?

*Empathy*

*Avoiding confrontation early about unnecessary test request*

P: Yes.

D: Firstly the kind of headaches you are experiencing aren't usually associated with brain tumours. I understand why people often worry about that though. Secondly you've had a CT scan which was entirely normal and this is very reassuring. You're entirely right in saying MRI can pick up very small abnormalities in the brain that CTs don't, but such tiny abnormalities would not cause these headaches. So going down the line of waiting for an MRI might give you reassurance but will not solve these headaches for you.

*Explanation according to ideas and concerns*

*Appropriately pitched for this patient using similar language she has used*

P: OK, I understand.

D: Apart from a tumour, have you any other ideas why you might be getting them?

Exploring ideas

P: One doctor said it may be my eyes. So I got them checked, and they were fine. I just feel like everything is quite stressful at the moment.

D: You say everything is quite stressful, what is exactly going on?

Picking up cue with open question

P: Well I'm studying law at the moment and I have a lot of exams and assignments. When these headaches come on I can't sit in front of the computer, I just have to go and lie down. It makes it much harder for me.

D: Yes I can see that it must be quite hard for you. How long do you study for at a time?

Empathy

P: It varies, I can do all nighters before my exams, but usually it's about 15 hours a day.

D: That is a long time. Do you get any other symptoms like neck pain?

Appropriate use of closed questions

P: Not really, I get some pain around my eyes but that's it really.

D: How are your exam preparations going?

P: Not good at all, I think it's because when I do try and work I think about these headaches. It's not good at all.

D: You are working a lot of hours a day. Is there a reason for that, are you behind or trying to catch up for any reason?

P: I go to a very good university and the course is quite intense. I know I usually have to work a bit harder than everyone else. I don't just want to pass – I want to do well. I have set a lot of pressure on myself.

D: I totally understand that. I would think that your headaches are being caused by the stress you are under. People who have headaches due to stress are called tension headaches. Have you heard of that before?

Explanation
Checking prior knowledge of condition

P: I think I've heard that from one of the other doctors.

D: In a way it means tension in terms of stress but it's referring to the tension built up in the scalp muscles. People describe those headaches in the same way you have. This is important to consider as we need to alleviate the reasons for the tension. Commonly people get them when they are stressed, due to hunched shoulders and working too hard. So we need to consider your working pattern. Have you thought about taking more breaks when you work?

Exploring causes of headaches

P: Yeah maybe I will consider that now, instead of just trying to work through the pain. It usually just gets worse.

D: Do you get much exercise?

P: Not recently, I should do more I know.

D: I think it is quite important. At the end of the day, it's the quality of the work that is important. Taking breaks just to stretch or get some fresh air will really help. Also setting parameters – it's not really right to work through the night; you will just get more tired. You can also consider painkillers, such as paracetamol or ibuprofen, but I imagine you've tried them all?

Formulating a solution with patient

P: Yes, they never work

D: Well, old-fashioned antidepressants aren't often used for depression these days but are used for tension headaches. We could consider that. It may be best to see if we can manage this with some changes to your lifestyle and then if you come back to me in a few weeks? I know you mentioned the neurologist, but I'm quite certain that they won't be able to help any more. I don't want you to be waiting a few months for them to say the same thing.

Organising follow-up

P: No, that's fine I will try reducing my stress and will come back to you in a few weeks. Thanks.

## Patient scenario 4

| Transcript | Skills demonstrated |
|---|---|
| **D:** Hello Mr Cavanagh. Come in. How can I help today?<br><br>**P:** Well I'm much the same to be honest. | Used patient's name<br>Open question |
| **D:** OK, I do have your notes here but would you mind telling me what's been going on?<br><br>**P:** Is it not in my notes? | Open question |
| **D:** Yes it is but we haven't met before and so it can be very helpful to hear everything from your perspective?<br><br>**P:** OK, I've still got pain. The doctor said it's tennis elbow but I don't play tennis – I mean I know you don't have to play tennis to have tennis elbow and I've had a look on the internet – it seems like it's what I've probably got. Paracetamol is not helping and nor is ibuprofen. I'm kind of struggling at the moment. The doctor says to rest but how do you rest your arm? | Explaining need to recap |
| **D:** Yes it sounds like it's been very difficult for you. Just to clarify, you have seen a few doctors here and you are happy with the diagnosis of tennis elbow?<br><br>**P:** Yes – it is exactly as they said, and from what I've been reading.<br><br>**D:** OK, good. Could I just confirm which arm is affected?<br><br>**P:** It's my right arm.<br><br>**D:** And are you right handed?<br><br>**P:** Yes, that's right.<br><br>**D:** So at the moment we have tried the painkillers, has there been anything else?<br><br>**P:** Yes, tried the painkillers and I've been referred to the physio. I know they said there would be a bit of a wait but I've been waiting for 4 weeks already and I'm really struggling. | Empathy<br>Clarifying |
| **D:** OK, before we talk a bit more about what we can do for you could you explain the pain a bit more to me? | Signposting and open question |

**P:** It's an ache, if I do certain movements it hurts more. I knocked it the other day and it was absolute agony.

**D:** Does it affect your sleep?

*Exploring impact of illness*

**P:** Not really, but I'm just frustrated at work and at home.

**D:** What do you do for a living?

*Picking up cue*

**P:** I'm a plasterer, so resting is not really an option.

**D:** No, that is difficult. Can you tell me how it is affecting you at work?

**P:** Well I'm working a lot more slowly than usual, I don't think I'm getting the perfect finish I usually do and I keep having to take breaks. I think the contractors think I'm lazy. This isn't a good time to be working slowly or not doing a good job – there isn't a huge amount of work available.

**D:** Well it sounds like a very stressful time. I'm sorry that the things we have tried haven't been working. Do you work for a company or are you self-employed?

*Empathy*

**P:** I work for myself so I lose money if I don't work.

**D:** That is difficult and I understand why you are frustrated that treatments don't seem to be working. You also mentioned things are difficult at home.

*Reflecting back and picking up earlier cues*

**P:** It's just the finances – I haven't been taking on as much work as I'd like to. You know I have a young family, and if I don't work we don't pay the mortgage.

**D:** Has it got to the stage where you are having financial worries?

**P:** It's getting there, not there yet but if it carries on like this it will.

**D:** Is this something you wanted to talk about in a bit more detail or get help or advice about?

*Clarifying expectations*

**P:** No, it's OK. I'm just about OK. But if I do I can come back.

D: I know that you mentioned doing some reading on tennis elbow. Is there anything you've read that you would like to discuss, or have you got any thoughts on what you would like to happen from here?

**Exploring expectations**

P: Well the last doctor mentioned an injection which sounds like it may help and obviously the physio, which I'm still waiting for.

D: Yes, they are all completely reasonable suggestions and I think from what you've told me today I really think we need to get you get back to normal. I also think what you do for a living is probably making the situation worse, as the constant movement will be causing more inflammation. I'm very sorry about the waiting time for the physio, what I could do is to try giving them a call and see if they can see you sooner, especially if it is affecting work.

**Showing understanding and that you have been listening**

**Coming up with solution**

P: That would be great.

D: How do you feel about the injection?

P: I'd rather do physio first and then the injection after if it doesn't work.

D: Sure, can you take me through the painkillers you are on now?

P: I'm taking probably about eight paracetamol a day and about two ibuprofens a day but the ibuprofen doesn't work.

D: OK, why don't we try a topical ibuprofen, which may be more helpful particularly as it's a specific area that is hurting? I think you're doing the right thing with a paracetamol so don't stop that, but I think maybe we should consider a stronger anti-inflammatory such as naproxen. It will just take the edge off the pain and may help you while we wait for the physio. Is there anything else that is worrying you?

P: No, I think everything you suggested sounds good.

D: It's just important to clarify I few things before I prescribe the naproxen. Do you suffer with asthma, indigestion, or have you ever had a stomach ulcer?

**Appropriate closed questioning when exploring contraindications**

**P:** No.

**D:** OK, that's fine. Taken the naproxen twice a day with food and if you get any problems, particularly indigestion, stop it and let me know. Why don't you give me a call next week and then I can update you with the physio appointment and you can let me know how the topical ibuprofen and naproxen is working out?

**P:** OK, thanks.

| | Safety netting |
| --- | --- |
| | Organising follow-up |

## Patient scenario 5

| Transcript | Skills demonstrated |
| --- | --- |
| **D:** Hello Mrs Nicholls. Please have a seat. | Used patient's name |
| **P:** Thank you. | |
| **D:** How are you? | |
| **P:** I'm OK – I've just come in for my review appointment, I saw your colleague a few weeks ago and did some tests because of the pain in my joints. | |
| **D:** That's right, I do have your notes here but since we haven't met before would you mind recapping what has been happening? | Exploring a patient's understanding and prior knowledge |
| **P:** So for the last 10 months I've just been having these pains in my hands and sometimes my wrists and elbows, in the morning. I feel like I have to get them going a bit and loosen them up – they really are quite painful. | |
| **D:** OK, when you spoke to my colleague did you discuss what could be going on? | |
| **P:** She mentioned that it could be rheumatoid arthritis or something horrible like that. So I'm obviously just hoping it's not that. | |
| **D:** So you mentioned rheumatoid arthritis. The tests that my colleague did, along with the examination of your joints and the history you gave, do indicate that you are suffering from rheumatoid arthritis. | Giving results clearly |

P: Oh God, really? I can't believe it. I was hoping you were going to say something else.

D: I know this must be very difficult news for you [*silence follows for 15 seconds*].

Empathy and use of silence

P: Does that mean I definitely do?

D: I think with the symptoms you have described and the test results I do think that this is the case. [*Pause.*]

Honesty and sensitivity

D: Would you mind telling me what you know about rheumatoid arthritis?

Exploring prior knowledge of condition

P: It's just a horrible disease, my grandma had it and she was really sick. I think she had something wrong with her chest as well. She was in a wheelchair. I just remember her having these horrible hands and my grandad had to do everything for her ... [*Pause.*]

P: Oh no, this is terrible. How long before my hands go like my grandma's?

D: I can understand why you are upset. The first thing to understand is that treatments have changed since your grandma's time. We have very good treatments that prevent specific changes that occur in the joints. It sounds like your grandma had very bad rheumatoid arthritis but there's no reason to suspect that you will get that way.

Empathy and giving reassurance based on concerns

P: And you can't tell me that I won't for sure?

D: It is always very difficult to give guarantees but treatment really has come on a long way.

P: So what do I do?

D: Well I think at the moment the important thing is to talk about the diagnosis and what that means for you, and then maybe we can talk about possible treatments. You are obviously and understandably very shocked. [*Pause.*] Do you have any questions for me?

Signposting
Giving patient space and time to think

P: Do you think I've got this because my grandma had it?

**D:** Rheumatoid arthritis is not an inherited condition, so that means it's not passed from one person to another but I think it tends to occur more in some families than others. It is not something I know an enormous amount about and I'd have to look into that for you to be able to give you any more information. Is there anything you are concerned about?

Explanation with appropriately pitched language
Phrase to explain lack of knowledge in an area; handling questions when you don't know the exact answer

**P:** Well I have a little girl, so I'm worried she may get it. Is there anything I can do to prevent her from getting it?

**D:** The first thing is that there really isn't anything to say that she will get it – in fact she is much more likely not to be affected, and there isn't anything you could really do to prevent it.

**P:** OK, oh dear, I don't know what I'm going to tell my husband.

**D:** What are you worried about?

Exploring concerns

**P:** I just don't know how he will handle it; I can't see him doing for me what my grandad did for my grandma. He's always working, he's always so busy.

**D:** As I say treatments are different now. It's not anything that is likely to happen any time soon. We run support groups and you are very welcome to come in and speak to the specialist rheumatoid arthritis nurse. What do you do for a living?

Offering reassurance and support

**P:** I play the violin professionally and I teach.

**D:** How have you been managing to do that?

Exploring impact of diagnosis on life

**P:** You know – as I said in the morning it's painful so I've started classes later in the day, but there are some days where it's quite hard. I have noticed that it's getting more difficult to play.

**D:** If you had to stop playing, how would you survive financially?

**P:** Financially I don't think it would be too bad, as my husband has a very good job. I do this more for enjoyment. It's a great passion of mine and I can't imagine not playing to be honest.

| | |
|---|---|
| **D:** I can understand this must be quite upsetting and a lot to take in. You will undoubtedly have a lot of questions. Perhaps I could give you some information of support groups and online resources where you can read a bit more on rheumatoid arthritis. Then we can arrange to meet again to discuss treatment? | Showing understanding<br><br>Information leaflets<br>Support groups |
| **P:** Yes, I think that would be best, I don't think I could take in any more information today. | |
| **D:** OK, we'll make an appointment to see me again in a few weeks. If you have any more questions in the meantime then I'll give you the number for our specialist nurse. Otherwise I'll see you in a few weeks time. | Organising follow-up |
| **P:** OK, thanks. | |

## Patient scenario 6

| Transcript | Skills demonstrated |
|---|---|
| **D:** Good morning Mrs Jameson. Come in. | Used patient's name |
| **P:** So I've just been told that you've lost my tests results, have you lost my sample or just the results? [*angry*] | |
| **D:** OK, I've only just found out about this now and I would just like to say I am also quite shocked about it. | Dealing with anger |
| **P:** I can tell you now that you are not as shocked or as angry as I am. This is absolutely disgusting and I cannot believe this has happened. | |
| **D:** I can totally understand why you are upset. I would be too if I were in your position. If I could try and talk through what has happened with the enquiries I have made? | Empathy |
| **P:** You can try but I doubt it will make anything better. So what did happen? | |
| **D:** So, you came in 3 weeks ago for the biopsy on your leg. The specimen we took was sent to the lab in the hospital. The specimen was due to be processed by experts at the hospital, where they look at it under the microscope. The hospital received the sample but somewhere along the line the sample has been lost. I've contacted them to ask why this has happened and they are looking into it, but I have no answers as yet. | Simple clear explanation |

P: Does this happen all the time or is this a one off?

D: I have never experienced this happening before and it is certainly unacceptable. I understand that, and we need to look into why this happened and prevent it from happening again.

*Understanding severity of error*

P: Well that doesn't help me at all; I've come in and wasted time, had quite a painful procedure and been worrying for the past few weeks, and then all to be told that the sample has been lost. Has someone tried looking for it? Or has someone just said 'oh well it's not here' but no one has bothered to look?

D: I can assure you that missing samples like this happen very infrequently and there will be an enquiry as to what has happened.

P: I want someone to take responsibility. It is absolutely unbelievable that this has happened. So what happens now, what if I have cancer on my leg? Who will take responsibility for that?

D: I totally understand why you are upset and frustrated; all I can do is offer my apologies for why this happened. I do not know why this happened and we will look into it. However, I do think it's important to look into what we can do next to help you with this lesion on your leg.

*Empathy – continues to maintain composure and offer explanation in face of angry patient*

P: Yes absolutely. Is someone going to do another biopsy now? What's the procedure from here?

D: OK, you mentioned before that you were worried about the possible diagnosis? What is it that you are very worried about?

*Reflecting back and exploring ICE*

P: Well obviously I'm worried that it's cancer and the thing is, the longer this takes the worse my chances will be. Everyone knows that with cancer you have to catch it early on.

D: OK, I can understand why you are very worried but if I can reassure you, we didn't take the biopsy because we think its cancer. We took the biopsy because your leg wasn't improving and we don't know what it is. We aren't specifically worried about cancer.

*Empathy and reassurance based on patient's concerns*

P: Well, how do you know?

D: Of course no one can be entirely sure, and that is a valid question. However, I do not suspect this is cancer. I know it doesn't help that we need to organise another biopsy and I know you mentioned that you have a difficult schedule to take time out.

*Reflecting back what the patient said earlier*

P: Exactly. I have no time to be coming in and out of the surgery, and appointments are hard to get.

D: Absolutely, we will try and find a time that would suit you to have it done as soon as we can.

*Demonstrating flexibility*

P: That's the least I would expect.

D: OK, so what time would suit you?

P: I work varying shifts, but I usually start at 9 am so could I come in at 8 am as soon as the practice opens? Could you not do it today?

D: I won't be able to do it today as I need a nurse here and I need to prepare all the equipment much like the first time you had this done. But we can certainly fit you in tomorrow morning if that suits you?

P: I guess that will have to do. How can I be sure that you won't lose my sample again?

D: All I can offer is my surprise that it happened in the first place. As I said this does happen very infrequently, I can't imagine it would happen again. I will ask them to process it urgently. I will look into why this has happened at all.

*Continuing to stay calm and offer to investigate formally*

P: Please do, as I don't want this happening to anyone else. The stress is unimaginable.

D: Yes, I completely understand. You mentioned that work is difficult, what do you do?

*Picking up cue*

P: I'm a cleaner; I have about five different houses that I go to.

D: Would you like me to write a letter saying that you will need to take time off?

*Offering help and a solution to the problem*

**P:** No, it's OK. I don't want anyone knowing, I'll figure something out.

**D:** Well if you come in tomorrow at 8.30 am and then we take the sample and then once we find out what this is we can discuss what to do next.

Organising follow-up

**P:** OK, thank you.

## Patient scenario 7

| Transcript | Skills demonstrated |
|---|---|
| **D:** Hello Mrs Armstrong, please come in and have a seat. My name is Dr Paul. | Used patient's name |
| **P:** Hello there. | |
| **D:** I know you have seen one of my colleagues before and have had a few investigations done, but as we have not met before I thought it would be a good idea if we could briefly discuss the symptoms you have been experiencing? | Recapping history and checking patient's understanding |
| **P:** Yes, OK. You've probably read this before but for the last 6 or 7 months I have been getting some crampy tummy pains. They have been happening whenever really – not every day although they can be every day at times. Sometimes I go without pain for about a week but then it comes back and I feel a bit bloated and sick. That's why Dr Smith sent me for some tests. | |
| **D:** Yes, absolutely. Was there anything you were specifically concerned about? | Exploring ICE |
| **P:** Well it's been on my mind for a while now and I have been really worried about things like cancer or something horrible going on as it has been quite painful at times. | |
| **D:** A lot of patients who are experiencing the same sort of symptoms as you are worried about cancer, and at this point I can reassure you that all your tests are normal. | Alleviating anxiety early |
| **P:** Oh, brilliant. OK. | |
| **D:** If we could just go through the tests? | Signposting |
| **P:** Yes, that would be great. | |

**D:** You had a blood test which showed no anaemia, so you have plenty of red blood cells, and the function of your kidneys and liver are completely normal. The colonoscopy, which is the test that you had done at the hospital ...

*Explaining results without using jargon*

**P:** Oh that one!

**D:** Yes. That one looked at the lining of the bowel and showed no problems whatsoever.

**P:** That's reassuring.

**D:** Yes that's very reassuring and I hope I can reassure you that from those investigations you don't need to be concerned about bowel cancer. That's effectively ruled out.

*Clear reassurance linked to previously expressed concerns*

**P:** That's great. So do you know if I need to do anything else or is there anything else that can tell me what it is?

**D:** Well, I have told you that most of these tests were normal but that's not solving the problem as you are still getting this pain. Maybe it would be a good idea now to move on to working out what it is and what can be done about it?

*Signposting a change of direction*

**P:** Yes.

**D:** The symptoms you are describing sound very much like irritable bowel syndrome to me. Is that something you have heard of before?

*Checking prior knowledge and understanding*

**P:** Well yes. Obviously I have been looking things up on the internet and that did come up as something I had thought about as it does fit with some of the things I have been experiencing. I did wonder whether I had that.

**D:** Would it be helpful if I talked a little bit about irritable bowel syndrome?

*Signposting*

**P:** Yes, very as I am not sure I understand it fully.

**D:** Well it's not particularly well understood but it's a condition with symptoms you have described – pain, bloating, sometimes loose stools, sometimes constipation. Some people feel various things make it worse and better. Have you yourself noticed anything that makes it worse?

**P:** Let me think – I suppose I have thought it may be something I am eating but I don't think that's the case as it just comes on regardless of what I've eaten. I do get it a lot more when I am at work than when I am at home. Actually, in the Christmas holidays it got a lot better when I was a bit more rested with more sleep.

**D:** What do you do for work?

Picking up on cue and exploring psychosocial factors

**P:** I'm a school teacher.

**D:** That must be quite busy?

**P:** Very.

**D:** And do you feel stressed?

**P:** Actually, I think I have been for the last few months. It's been a difficult time, not with work as such, but my mother's been put in a nursing home recently. She had to be placed there as she is a bit confused and has not been keeping that well. That's been on my mind and there are a few silly little things, like I keep getting called at work from the nursing home staff who leave messages about things like tablets and my mum. I obviously panic, but actually it's always been OK.

**D:** Well that must be really stressful for you?

**P:** Yes it is.

**D:** It must be very difficult when a relative has moved into a nursing home and having all those phone calls as well.

Empathy

**P:** Yes.

**D:** Is there anything you think could help with the stress or take some of it away?

Exploring patient's own ideas
Involving patient

**P:** I don't know. I haven't really thought about it, I panic. I suppose it would be helpful if they stopped calling me at work, as obviously I panic that something serious has happened when usually it's about the fact they need another prescription or are wondering about medications. If they stopped calling me that would help.

**D:** Right. Do you have any siblings who could share this responsibility?

**P:** No, it's just me.

**D:** That's quite a lot of responsibility.

| | Understanding support/ social situation |

**P:** Yes. I'm her next of kin.

**D:** It sounds as though a lot of the problems they are calling you about could be dealt with by the GP.

| | Empathy |

**P:** I wasn't aware that GPs deal with this sort of thing?

**D:** Yes absolutely. It sounds as though if they had some instructions and everything was made clearer, there may be no need for them to call you.

| | Offering solutions for the problem |

**P:** Right.

**D:** The other thing some people find helpful is to organise a time when the staff know that you are going in to visit, when you can get all the questions answered face-to-face once a week and all the minor things that don't really need to be spoken about immediately could be put on hold until then.

**P:** I could do that as I go every week, sometimes twice a week. Maybe I could tell them to wait and speak to me then unless it is an emergency. That might help.

**D:** Well I am pleased to reassure you that this is not bowel cancer, which I understand you were worried about. Stress does make irritable bowel syndrome worse, so maybe if we could deal with that then some of the things causing stress your symptoms would improve. If they don't, there are other things we can try. There are some medications that are quite useful.

| | Reflecting back |

**P:** Oh right.

**D:** And if diarrhoea becomes an issue there are other medications for that. So there are always things available that we could go to if we need to. Would you find it useful if I gave you an information leaflet?

| | Discussing options for future care and involving patient in management decisions |

**P:** Yes, that would be great, and the names of these tablets. Can I buy them?

**D:** You can get some of them over the counter but maybe it would be a good to meet in a couple of weeks time to see how you are getting on and whether you need to start any of these tablets.

Organising follow-up

**P:** It may be difficult in the next few weeks with exams coming up at school.

**D:** I know it's difficult for you to come in. We do evening surgeries – mine is on Thursdays and you are welcome to book into that. Alternatively we could do it by telephone as we are just talking about symptoms.

Showing understanding of primary care

**P:** You can do that? That would be very helpful as it saves me parking here. That would be great.

**D:** Shall I organise that and I'll leave the information leaflet at reception for you? If you think of any questions – often people leave and they think they should have asked something – then please call me. I may not be able to take the call but I will call you back. The same applies if any of your symptoms get worse or change in any way.

Follow-up and safety netting
Written information

**P:** Thank you.

## Patient scenario 8

| Transcript | Skills demonstrated |
|---|---|
| **D:** Hello Mrs White, I'm Dr Lewis. Come on in. | Used patient's name |
| **D:** How can I help? | Open question |
| **P:** I don't know if you've got any of the information about what's been going on in the last few weeks but I've come in today because I have had this thing with my leg that I went to hospital about. It became really painful on my right side. They told me that I had a DVT. | |
| **D:** Yes, that is right, can you tell me a bit more about this? | Open question – encouraging patient to tell her story |

P: They said that it can be serious and I need to be on treatment for the next few months. I've never had anything wrong with me and I'm going to hospital having all these blood tests and I'm on these tablets, and I really want to talk to you about what this is all about.

D: Of course, it must be quite a stressful time for you.

Empathy

P: Yes, you know I'm only 32 and I feel like an old woman taking all these tablets and I don't know if I really need them. What's going on? Is it going to come back?

D: OK, would you mind telling me about what you already know about the DVT and the medications?

Checking understanding

P: Well, there is nothing normally wrong with me but I just had this pain in my calf muscle and I was training for the marathon and I was running quite a lot but I stopped for a while and then it was really painful. So I went to the hospital because a friend told me to get it checked out and they said I had a clot in a vein and it was serious and I needed tests. And I think somebody mentioned that it was life threatening.

D: Yes, that must have been scary for you.

Empathy

P: It was and they asked me loads and loads of questions and you know they asked me if I smoked and obviously I don't do anything like that. Another thing they said was to stop the pill and they said that it might be related – but I've been on that for years, since I was 22 I think.

D: Had anything happened before that could have led to this? For example had you been ill before or been on any long journeys or flights?

Closed questioning

P: No, not that I can think of.

D: OK, would it be helpful if I just explained a bit about what has been going on?

Signposting change of direction

P: Yes, that would be good.

**D:** You unfortunately had a deep vein thrombosis and that really means a blood clot in a vein in your leg. In itself that isn't overly serious but occasionally those blood clots can break off and go into the lungs. This is called a pulmonary embolism, which can be a lot more serious and so this is the reason that you were started on medicines to thin the blood, to prevent any more clots. They also did some tests to see why this had happened, as in some cases you can find out the cause. For example, you may have an inherited condition that may make you more likely to have blood clots forming. But in most cases that isn't the case. No one really knows why it happens and that is the case with you, your tests were entirely normal.

**D:** You mentioned they stopped your pill and that's the right thing as one of the hormones in the pill can increase the risk of you getting blood clots. This is why we always ask when we prescribe the pill if you have had blood clots in the past.

**D:** So at the moment you are taking warfarin, how are you getting on with that?

**P:** I don't really like it to be honest, I have to keep taking time off to go to the hospital to have the blood tests and I just don't like it. First of all I don't like taking tablets, and then they keep changing my dose, and it is all very confusing. I would really prefer not be on them and that's part of why I've come in today. I want to know if it's something I really need to take as I feel much better now.

**D:** Well, I think you really do need to take it. There have been lots of studies done on people that have these types of blood clots that have shown that you will be safest if you take the warfarin for 3 months. I understand that having these blood tests is quite frustrating and disruptive, and I can only say that you are in the worst stage at the moment, because we have to work out the correct dosage you need. You will probably find that in a few weeks' time that you will only need to get the blood tests done every couple of weeks once everything has become more stable.

**P:** OK, well the other thing is after 3 months do I just stop it and is the DVT not going to come back?

Clear explanation pitched at appropriate level

Explanation

Empathy

**D:** When you have a blood clot you are at slightly higher risk of having another blood clot. The pill may well have contributed in your case and so that cause has now been removed. It may also be worth having a talk to the haematologist at the hospital, the doctor who runs the warfarin clinic, to see if they think it is important for you to take some sort of blood thinner before long haul flights or journeys. You also mentioned you have stopped the pill. What form of contraception are you using now?

Sexual health promotion

**P:** Nothing at the moment. I'm using condoms as I am so worried about hormonal stuff now.

**D:** Well there are other options we can go through that are safe for you, but I am aware time is short. Could we arrange another appointment to discuss this in more detail?

Managing time but picking up important related issues

**P:** That would be good. Oh, one other thing – what do you think about exercising and running? Will I be able to run the marathon? Can I carry on training?

**D:** Well, how are you feeling now?

**P:** Good! I feel much better now; no pain anymore, only a little redness around my leg. I would just be worried to continue if that was the cause.

**D:** When you have a blood clot, as you noticed, you get swelling in the leg, and I would have thought prolonged running would have made that worse, so I would probably advise against anything too serious at the moment. But I must say it's not something I've ever been asked before and so I will have to ask my colleagues at the hospital and get back to you about that one.

Verbalising thoughts but seeking expert opinion. Honest and open.

**D:** So, we have talked about quite a lot today and obviously it's a stressful time for you. You mentioned that your boss isn't happy about you going to these tests. What do you do for work?

Reflecting back and picking up cues

**P:** I work in advertising for a big company.

**D:** Would it help if I wrote to a letter to them to explain what has been going on?

**P:** Yes, that would be very useful, thank you.

D: OK, I'll do that and leave it at reception for you, along with an information leaflet on DVT and contraception, and if you think of anymore more questions let me know and we can discuss it next time. Also, once I've found out the information for your marathon training, I'll be in touch.

Providing written information and follow up

## Patient scenario 9

| Transcript | Skills demonstrated |
|---|---|
| D: Hi Mr Medland, do come in. | Used patient's name |
| D: How can I help? | Open question |
| P: I've just come back for my tests results. | |
| D: Of course, but before we go through all that can I just ask you to tell me a bit more about why these tests were done? | |
| P: Do you not have my notes? | |
| D: Yes I have, I've just had a quick read but it's the first time we've met, so if you don't mind explaining what has been going on it would help me to put everything into context. | Clear explanation |
| P: I've just been feeling absolutely exhausted, there must be something going on. I'm sleeping well but I'm constantly tired, I just have no energy to do anything. My wife said to come in and get checked out. Maybe I'm anaemic or something? Maybe I need some iron but basically the doctor said to do some tests and that's why I'm back. | |
| D: OK, how long have you been feeling like this? | Closed question |
| P: Well, for a couple of months I've been exhausted. | |
| D: OK, before we go on do you want me to go through all the tests we have done and give you the results? Then we can talk a little bit more about the problem. | Signposting and controlling the consultation
Explaining results clearly |
| P: Yes, OK. | |

**D:** So I understand you saw my colleague and he said to come back after the blood tests so we could rule out some of the causes of tiredness that we can potentially treat, for example you mentioned anaemia. We did the test for anaemia and we also checked your kidney, liver and thyroid function which could all cause feelings of tiredness. Fortunately all of these were completely normal, so I can reassure you that you don't need any iron tablets.

Linking reassurance to previously expressed ideas

**P:** Great.

**D:** But you are still feeling tired so I just want to ask you a few more questions. You mentioned it has been going on for a few months. Is there anything else that you have been feeling or any other symptoms?

Reflecting back

Open question

**P:** Not really, it's just, I get back home quite late and I just crash on the sofa with no energy to do anything really.

**D:** You mentioned that your wife was telling you to come here as it's something she has noticed as well, but do you have any thoughts about why you have been feeling like this for the last few months?

Exploring ideas

**P:** No, I guess it's stress but I sleep OK, you know I wake up and feel alright but a couple of hours later I feel exhausted again.

**D:** Would you mind if I asked you a few specific symptoms?

Signposting

**P:** That's fine

**D:** How is your mood generally?

Closed questions

**P:** OK, there is a lot going on but I'm not one of these people that get depressed.

**D:** How is your sleep?

**P:** I'm sleeping fine.

**D:** How many hours do you get?

**P:** Probably about 7 hours, I get home from work at 8 pm, a few hours to relax then sleep for about 7 hours.

D: You seem to be working late, is that a daily thing?

P: Yes, for the last few months.

D: What do you do for a living?

P: My main job is at a DIY shop. I'm a sales assistant but I also have another job that I do in the evening, four nights a week in the petrol station.

D: That sounds like you are doing a lot of hours in a short time. Is there anyone else at home apart from your wife? Any children?

P: No – just me and my wife. She lost her job 6 months ago so I'm trying to pick up the financial slack

D: I am sorry to hear that. You mentioned earlier that there is a lot going on – is there anything else that is affecting you?

P: My dad is ill at the moment. Well I say he is ill, I think he's just more old than ill. He lives alone since my mum died. I have to see him quite a lot so I pop in most evenings after work. I know he is always thinking I should be there more. I don't think he understands that I'm working hard. I think he's lonely.

D: It sounds like you have a lot of stress on you and pressure at the moment. Have you thought about anything that could help you?

P: Yes, maybe I think my wife should see my dad more often. But I guess it's good that my blood tests are fine. My wife will be pleased about that. She thought they wouldn't be.

D: Was there anything you or your wife was particularly worried about?

P: Not really, she thinks I drink too much but she is just being over-cautious – she thought it was my liver.

D: Do you mind me asking how much you do drink?

P: It's not that much, a few pints, just beer. I don't drink spirits.

---

Picking up on cues (and listening to a patient's responses)

Empathy
Picking up on cues

Empathy
Exploring ideas and expectations

Picking up on cues

D: On an average day how many pints would you say you are having?

P: I have about four or five a day.

D: OK, so that is a bit more than you should drink and your wife is obviously concerned about you. Is it something you have thought about cutting down on?

Health promotion

P: I just need to relax, you know. You get home late, put your feet up, have a couple of pints and put the day behind you.

D: I understand, but while you may find that drinking in the evenings helps you to relax, in the longer term it is probably contributing to your stress and fatigue and it really would be a good idea to reduce it. It sounds like you do have a lot going on and what you have told me today certainly explains your symptoms.

P: I was kind of hoping you would say 'it's your thyroid, take this and feel better'.

D: I can see how that would be easier for you. But it does sound like you are under a lot of pressure and strain with the hours you work and your dad. Have you discussed how you feel with your wife?

Empathy and dealing with psychosocial aspects

P: Yes, I have.

D: You haven't planned any time away, any holidays?

P: No, we don't have the time to do that right now.

D: I think it is really important that you try to tackle all of the stress. You are obviously working very hard and the need to see your father seems to be adding to your stress. Have you thought about speaking to him, maybe seeing whether he would attend a day group or something similar to help with his loneliness?

Discussing options to come up with a solution together

P: That is not a bad idea – I think I need to talk to him and only go over a few times a week. Maybe my wife could take him out during the days as well.

D: That sounds like a very good idea. You have certainly got a lot going on. Maybe we should see you again in a few weeks just to touch base on your stress and your alcohol. But if you need to come in and speak to us earlier then please do.

Organising follow up

P: Thank you.

## Patient scenario 10

| Transcript | Skills demonstrated |
|---|---|
| D: Good afternoon Mr Livesey, please come in. | Used patient's name |
| D: How can I help you today? | Open question |
| P: I don't think there is much you can do to be honest, my girlfriend said to come down. I'm struggling to sleep and things like that. | |
| D: OK, would you mind telling me a little bit more. | Open question |
| P: I've been struggling for a while. There has been a lot going on, I think I know what it is. I think it's just one of those things time will make better. | |
| D: Would you like to tell me what you think is causing these problems? | Open question – encouraging patient to tell their story |
| P: Well I used to be in the Army. It was good but I had some pretty traumatic things happen when I was on tour. At first you just try and put it to the back of your mind. I think I have realised that it is always going to be with me. The thoughts of it always keep me up at night. | |
| D: Do you feel able to tell me more about these memories? | Open question |
| P: Yes, the main thing is that when we were on tour one of my troop was killed by a roadside bomb. | |
| D: I'm very sorry to hear that. | Empathy |
| P: Hmm, it was difficult, I get flashbacks of the event and of the next half hour of dealing with him. It is always there really. In the daytime I'm OK, although I feel it's always with me. But at night I wake up, I can't sleep. | |

**D:** It sounds like it was horrendous for you and I can understand why you are having problems now. When did it start affecting you?

Empathy

**P:** I got back 9 months ago, the Army has given us counselling. Actually more like a debrief, just a talk about what has happened. It was all right. I just thought things would get better with time. I thought everyone had been through the same and I would get past it. I really thought I would be better by now.

**D:** At this point I just want to reassure you that this is very common with people who have been through situations like you have. And it's very much suggestive of a condition called post-traumatic stress disorder or PTSD. Is this something you've heard of?

Reassurance and encouragement and checking prior knowledge

**P:** Yes, the Army mentioned that.

**D:** Is it every night that you experience flashbacks?

**P:** No, not every night.

**D:** And you mentioned your girlfriend asked you to come in, is she aware of what has been going on?

Reflecting back

**P:** Yes, I think sometimes I wake her up in the middle of the night. I think she is just fed up now. She keeps saying I should be sorting it out but I keep thinking it will go away and it hasn't.

**D:** Have you had any thoughts about how you would like to go about sorting things out?

Exploring expectations

**P:** I suppose some sort of therapy would be OK.

**D:** I agree. I do think it is important for you to have some psychological therapy and certain types can be very effective at treating PTSD.

**P:** Yes, I think that will be good.

**D:** Is it affecting you on a day-to-day basis?

Exploring impact on work/relationships

**P:** Yes, to a degree, but I'm getting on fine to be honest. I have a job and its fine – I work in recruitment now. I just think for my girlfriend's sake I need to sort it out.

D: Is it putting much strain on the relationship?

P: Yes, it is I guess, these things do, it's easy to bury your head in the sand.

D: How is your mood?

P: I'm fine, I'm not depressed or anything.

D: Are you eating well and managing to work during the day?

P: Yes, I'm doing OK, I just feel guilty about it happening in the first place. You know it's drilled into you that you have to look after your troop but I think I'm over that now. It's just these flashbacks.

D: How would you like to proceed?

Involving patient in treatment decisions

P: Just want your advice to be honest; I didn't know there was anything that could be done.

D: Maybe we can start by referring you to the psychologist to see what they suggest in the first instance. But we are also here as GPs, if things are getting stressful and you are finding it hard to sleep. We can give you some medications if you are feeling very anxious. Would it be helpful if I gave you just a bit of information on the condition itself and the treatment options and then you can think about where you want to go from there? And then if you come back and see me in a couple of weeks we can discuss it further?

Providing written information

Organising follow-up

P: Yes, that sounds like a good idea, thank you.

## Patient scenario 11

| Transcript | Skills demonstrated |
|---|---|
| D: Hello Mrs Jones, I'm Dr Smith. Please come in. | Used patient's name |
| D: How can I help? | Open question |
| P: Erm, yes … I don't know how to say it but I'm just worried about my gut actually. | |

D: OK, do you want to tell me a little bit more about what has been concerning you?

Open question

P: Well, it's just you see all these adverts on the TV and I'm just a bit worried really.

D: It is always a good idea to get things checked out. What has been going on?

Open question – keep trying to get the patient to tell you her story

P: Oh, it's a bit embarrassing really. It's just when I go to the toilet it's a little bit different than what it is like usually.

D: No, not at all, you've done the right thing by coming in. If we could go into a bit more detail? Could you tell me what has changed?

Reassurance and encouragement

P: Oh gosh it sounds embarrassing; it's very hard to talk about. I just have really bad diarrhoea. I've never had such loose stools before.

D: When did this start?

P: It's hard to pinpoint when, but easily over 3 or 4 months now.

D: Have you noticed anything else that has been worrying you?

Open question

P: Well, my clothes feel a lot looser now. I haven't got scales at home and I haven't weighed myself in years, but I used to be quite a plump lady but now I need to wear a belt with my trousers. Sometimes I get blood in my stools. So sorry to have to tell you this.

D: You have done the right thing by coming in. You mentioned you have seen the adverts on the TV?

Reflecting back

P: Yes, they always worry you, don't they.

D: What is it in the advert that has worried you?

Exploring ideas and concerns

P: I saw an advert that said blood in the stools can mean cancer, but I'm sure it's not that.

D: OK, well first we need to look into why this is happening. Would you mind if I asked you some specific questions?

Signposting

**P:** Go ahead.

**D:** You mentioned you have blood in the stool, what colour is the blood?

Closed questions

**P:** It varies really, sort of a brownish reddish blood.

**D:** Have you ever noticed that your motions are black in colour?

**P:** Not really, they are more sort of ... Oh gosh, this is very embarrassing. There's dark blood mixed in with the motions.

**D:** Please do not feel embarrassed. You mentioned your stools are very loose, more like diarrhoea?

Reassuring patient to encourage contribution

**P:** Yes, sometimes – but then sometimes I don't go for a few days and then I get diarrhoea.

**D:** Is there anything in your diet or home circumstances that has changed that could have caused the weight loss?

**P:** Well, my circumstances have definitely changed in the last year ... My husband is no longer with us. You know we used to cook together and have nice meals and now I guess I don't eat as much.

**D:** I am sorry to hear that. OK well, you have absolutely done the right thing by coming here. Some of the things you are describing make me concerned that something may be happening in the bowel. You mentioned bowel cancer and that is something we certainly need to rule out. This doesn't mean that you have bowel cancer but it is best to rule it out. Have you read about any of the tests we tend do for that sort of thing?

Empathy

Clear explanation

Checking prior knowledge

**P:** I've heard about that thing where they put a camera inside which sounds horrible and I don't really want to do that. Is there something you can do here? I really don't want to go to the hospital.

**D:** In the practice we would want to take some blood tests, but regardless of the blood tests results I think it would be wise to have further investigation that would be done at the hospital. Is there any reason you don't want to go to the hospital?

Picking up on cues

P: It's just my poor Henry, I took him into the hospital after his sudden collapse and then he died so quickly and now every time I walk past the hospital I just shudder. I couldn't even bring myself to visit my sister when she was ill in hospital last year. So I really don't want to go to hospital – it would just bring everything back.

D: I can understand that, it's common for patients to feel that way but I really do think it is important to have these tests; maybe we can look at sending you to a different hospital. The investigation that you've read about is called a colonoscopy and it's probably the best test but if you are finding it difficult to come to terms with it there are other tests such as a CT scan. This is something you can discuss with the consultant.

Empathy

P: Yes, well, if you think the tests are really important I guess there isn't anything else I can do.

D: If I can just recap what has been going on, and if I miss anything let me know and then we will talk about the next step. So, essentially, you have experienced a change in your bowel habit for the past couple of months. You've noticed loose motions and blood in the stool and that your clothes are looser now. You've done absolutely the right thing by coming in. We do need to investigate this. We will try and refer you to a different hospital and then see if they can do a CT in the first instance. Now I would like to do a blood test, also I will refer you to a hospital and you should hear from them in 2 weeks. If you don't then please contact the practice. If you have any questions in the meantime then just give us a call.

Summarising

Safety netting

P: Thank you.

## Patient scenario 12

| Transcript | Skills demonstrated |
|---|---|
| **D:** Hi Sophie, I am Dr Rahman. Come in. | Used patient's name |
| **D:** How are you? | Open question |
| **P:** I'm not bad, so I've got this letter from the housing department and the thing is I need you to write me a letter. | |
| **D:** OK, could you tell me a bit more about this? | Open question |
| **P:** The problem is, you know I'm having a baby. Well I'm 20 weeks. Well anyway, the baby is coming in a couple of months and so the council have said that I have to move to the other side of the city and you see – I've got to stay in this area because my mum is here. I've no idea where the dad is – he's just gone off and I have to have this baby on my own. Well basically, the council have said that if I have a complication with my pregnancy then I can stay here. So you know how I was on antibiotics last week can you just write me a letter and just say that I have had a complicated pregnancy and so the council will let me keep my place? | |
| **D:** Where do you live now? | Continuing to gather information rather than tackle request too early in consultation |
| **P:** I live with my mum. But I've applied to get my own place. There isn't any room at my mum's because there's too many of us in her house already. I can't be with my mum under the same roof too long as she does my head in but I will want her help with babysitting. | |
| **D:** You mentioned that there are too many people at your mum's already – who else is living with there? | Exploring social situation |
| **P:** Yes, my little sister who is 4 and my brother who is 8, I think. There is also my mum's boyfriend and my boyfriend was staying with us too but he's disappeared off now. Can you believe it, I'm having his baby and he left? | |
| **D:** That must be very difficult for you. Do you have any contact with him? | Empathy |
| **P:** No, I don't even want him around anymore, I don't care. | |
| **D:** It must all be very stressful for you and I can understand why you want your mother near you. Do you know where they are planning to move you to? | |

P: Yes, they said some place called Upminster I think. You can't even get one bus to my mum's from there – you have to change or take tubes and that.

D: Yes, that would be difficult for you. I can fully appreciate that you want to be near your mother and you would benefit from the support.

Empathy and support

P: Thanks, you understand what I have been thinking.

D: Do you have any friends that could help?

P: I had loads of friends, yeah, but they all just want to go out and party and I like that too, but I haven't been able to and so I haven't seen them in ages. But I've got some mates down the pool where I work.

D: What is it that you do?

P: I was a lifeguard yeah, but since I got pregnant and that, I work at the reception desk now.

D: You mentioned earlier that you were advised that if you had complications in the pregnancy they wouldn't move you. Who was it that gave you that advice?

Reflecting back

P: The council and someone at Citizens Advice.

D: Well, I agree with you, when you are in the later stages of your pregnancy that you would benefit from having your mother around to support you. I don't have any sway with Housing but I'm very happy to write to them and say that you it would help if you were near to your mother for support and guidance as a single mother. I can't say that you've had a complicated pregnancy. I know you had an infection that needed antibiotics but that wouldn't be classed as a complicated pregnancy at all. I would have to write a letter detailing the social reasons why you need to stay near your mother.

Empathy

Coming up with a solution/compromise

Being open and honest

P: I already told them everything but they said it had to be a medical problem. And it was a medical problem.

D: I can write what happened but they won't take that as a complication in pregnancy. They mean people who have been in and out of hospital with lots of medical problems.

P: Well could you say that I had lots of medical problems?

D: No, I won't be able to lie.

Probity

P: I had to go into the hospital for a scan because they were worried about the weight, is that not a complication?

D: I'm afraid there is no way as a professional I could or would lie to help you get housing. I'm very happy to support your request with what we've discussed but there is no way I could make anything up or exaggerate anything.

P: OK, well, if that's all you can do. Can I pick up the letter this afternoon?

D: It won't be ready this afternoon, probably in a few days.

P: Well, I need to take it the guy at the council tomorrow morning.

D: OK, I'll try and get it done for then. Is everything else OK with the pregnancy?

Showing flexibility and compromising with patient

P: Yeah I suppose. I felt the baby move the other day.

D: Have you got any other concerns?

P: No, not really, I just can't be away from my mum.

D: Of course. Could I just ask whether you smoke?

Health promotion

P: Yeah I smoke, but I'm now better though, because you told me before that I had to cut down. So I only smoke about 10 now, before I was smoking about 20.

D: Yes, do you know why we ask people to stop smoking?

P: Yes, because it hurts the baby.

D: Yes, you mentioned earlier that you had a scan because the doctors were worried about the baby's weight and smoking can affect the baby's growth. Have you thought about cutting back some more?

Picking up on cues, reflecting back

**P:** Yes, it's just you know when I'm stressed, like with this thing with the council, I just need to smoke.

**D:** No, I understand that it is hard, but I don't think you should give up on stopping smoking. Maybe you should see the nurse here that does the smoking cessation clinics.

Empathy and offering support with smoking cessation

**P:** OK, I'll do that.

**D:** How about your alcohol?

**P:** I've had the odd drink, but I've been really good. My mum keeps telling me not to drink and I don't go out that much anymore with my mates. So I probably have a couple of beers a week. So I've not really had that much.

**D:** Well, again, it's very important that alcohol is kept to a minimum. I think a small glass of wine or a small beer is OK once in a while but ideally it would be best to cut it out completely.

**P:** Yes, I'll try and you know I don't smoke any dope or anything anymore.

**D:** That is really good, well done for that. Just keep working on the cigarettes and alcohol, OK?

Encouraging and non-judgemental

**P:** OK thanks, and I can get the letter tomorrow, yeah?

**D:** Yes, it will be ready then.

**P:** Thanks.

# Patient scenario 13

| Transcript | Skills demonstrated |
|---|---|
| **D:** Hello Miss Carter, my name is Dr Jones. How can I help? | Used patient's name |
| **P:** Hi, I just wanted to have a chat with you about everything that has been going on. I don't know if you know what happened to me last week? | |
| **D:** Yes, I got a discharge letter from the eye casualty department. | |
| **P:** You know all of that happened and now I'm in this situation where I'm waiting and they've told me that I've got this thing in my eye that has caused all these problems. I just wanted to see if you could get me to see the neurologist a bit quicker. | |
| **D:** I have got a summary of what happened but would you mind just recapping in your own words what exactly has happened? | Checking patient's knowledge |
| **P:** You know last week I was at work and I just suddenly couldn't see out of my left eye properly, it was really frightening. So I told a colleague of mine who took me to eye casualty. A doctor had a look and they said that I had some sort of inflammation of my eye and then gave me some information. They said it is called optic neuritis. They said I needed a scan and they couldn't tell me what it was caused by and they said I have to see a neurologist and have an MRI. For me this is all so worrying, I can't really wait. | |
| **D:** I can appreciate this must be very stressful. Is there anything in particular that you are you worried about? | Empathy and exploring ICE |
| **P:** I went home and looked up all the things they said, I read about multiple sclerosis and that sounds horrible. I need to know what's wrong with me. | |
| **D:** I understand this must be a stressful time. How are the symptoms now? | Empathy and open question |
| **P:** I'm much better now, it hasn't happened again. But I'm always worried it's going to come back because they told me it's all inflamed. | |

**D:** Have you ever had any other funny symptoms in the past before all of this happened?

**P:** You know when I come to think of it I've had this weird time when my foot went numb – I just felt like I was walking on cotton wool for about a week or so. I didn't feel like I was walking properly. I kept telling people, but it was a few years ago. But nothing wrong with my eye before.

**D:** OK, you mentioned that you were worried about MS, what do you know about that?

Checking knowledge and understanding

**P:** I know that it's a condition that basically means you can lose your ability to see. Its nerve problem that can get worse and worse, and you end up in a wheelchair.

**D:** Well, MS has a variety of presentations. It's also a step too far to be worrying too much about MS at the moment; you have been diagnosed with optic neuritis which is a specific condition to the eye. Although it is true that this could possibly be a sign of MS, in many people it isn't, it's a one-off event that doesn't occur again. Obviously I can't give you any guarantees, but we will know more when you have the tests done.

Reassurance (as much as is possible)

Clear explanation

**P:** It's just the not knowing that is hard. If I know what is wrong then I can make provisions for me and my daughter. I just feel like I can't wait this long for a scan.

**D:** Have you heard anything about the appointments?

**P:** I have an appointment for the MRI this week and then with the neurologist the following week.

**D:** I understand that it is very hard for you at the moment; I'll try and see if I can bring the hospital appointment forward. You mentioned you were worried about your little girl. What's the situation at home?

Empathy

**P:** Well it's just us two at home, she's only 3. Its hard work now her dad's gone. I do have a few friends who help me out when I have to work late and everything.

**D:** I'm sorry to hear that. It sounds very stressful. What do you do?

Picking up on cue

P: I'm a sales manager.

D: OK, what does that involve?

P: I work in a shop but I'm a manager so I have to work late, especially with all the sales on at the moment.

D: And are you managing to cope at the moment – with all this stress and uncertainty going on?

Exploring impact of stress on home/work

P: It is hard. I am very distracted at work. I am thinking of asking whether I can reduce my hours for a few weeks.

D: That sounds very sensible. If you need any help to do that I would be happy to write you a note.

Support

P: Thank you – that would be very useful.

D: I know we have talked about quite a lot today – would you mind if I just recapped a few things?

P: That's fine.

D: Essentially you went to eye casualty after you had loss vision in the left eye where they diagnosed optic neuritis. Obviously you became concerned that it might be MS. Most people with optic neuritis don't develop MS, but it is a possibility. The next step is to have the MRI and then see the consultant. I'll try and bring the appointment forward but I can't guarantee this. In the meantime, if you have new symptoms then please let me know immediately. If you need anything for work then let me know. Would you prefer if I contact you by telephone once I find out what's going on with your appointment?

Summarising

Follow-up plan

P: Yes, that would be great, thank you.

## Patient scenario 14

| Transcript | Skills demonstrated |
|---|---|
| **D:** Good Morning Miss Jackson, I am Dr Lee. How may I help? | Uses patient's name and open question |
| **P:** Dr Thompson had said to me before about my colitis and he said I might need surgery. It's all just a bit of a shock really and I just want to have a chat about it. He told me yesterday and it's obviously the worst time for this to be happening. | |
| **D:** OK, why don't you tell me what you understand to be happening and then I can try to fill in the gaps. | Establishing understanding |
| **P:** So, Dr Thompson and I go back a long way. I had this colitis diagnosed a few years ago. I was getting bloody diarrhoea and I had bad pains. Everything was fine but then I had another bout of pains and bloody diarrhoea and I've had a few tests and now they say I might have to have an operation and may be left with a bag. I really don't think I can handle a bag. It's all too much really. | |
| **D:** It must be very upsetting and frightening. | Empathy |
| **P:** Yes. It has been a massive shock. | |
| **D:** How have you been feeling since Dr Thompson spoke to you? | |
| **P:** Well, my tummy feels better. I'm taking my steroids and everything. But Dr Thompson just said all these things to me and I've just been thinking about it and now I have all these questions. | |
| **D:** Did Dr Thompson talk to you about the surgery? | Checking understanding |
| **P:** To be honest, after he said there was a chance I'd have to have a bag, I just stopped listening. I know he said I may not need one but I'm feeling a bit pessimistic. | |
| **D:** Well, I can talk to you in general terms as to why we do surgery. As for specific details I'd have to ask Dr Thompson to go through that with you. Would that be helpful? | Managing expectations according to ability |
| **P:** Yes – that would be good. | |

**D:** Hopefully I'll be able to answer some of your questions.

**P:** Yes, please do.

**D:** Most of the time if there is an area of bowel that has too much disease, it becomes difficult to treat with medicine and we will remove that part and then sew it back together. But if during surgery it is too difficult to re-join the bowel we use a stoma and then a few months down the line we will remove the bag and then try and re-join the bowel.

*Appropriately pitched explanation*

**P:** Oh God, I can't even handle a bag for a few months. I really can't ...

**D:** Yes, it must be very hard. You mentioned earlier that this is the worst possible time for this to be happening. Can I ask why?

*Picking up on cues and reflecting back*

**P:** Well, work has just been so hectic at the moment. I've got my laptop with me now actually, as I'm just trying to get it all done. And also I'm getting married in the summer and the thing is my boyfriend doesn't really know what's been going on. To be honest I don't think he will want to marry a girl with a stoma, I just don't think he will.

**D:** I know it's very stressful for you.

*Empathy*

**P:** I don't know ... Do you think it's something that I've done that has made this happen?

**D:** Well, as you probably know with colitis it can just flare up for no real reason. You've previously been quite stable on the medicine – was there anything you thought could have caused this?

*Picking up on cues and exploring ideas*

**P:** Yeah it's been alright – I was on those tablets. But there have been times when I've felt really good so I haven't taken my medications. I didn't tell Dr Thompson this; you know what he's like. Do you think that's why?

**D:** I think it's always important to carry on taking the medicines but I can't say if that's why it's happened. Certainly in future you should try and take all of the medicine.

*Non-judgemental*

P: I just feel really rubbish now. If I had taken the medication I probably wouldn't be in this mess, especially before my wedding.

D: Try not to worry about that at the moment. You are here now and we just need to deal with this situation as best we can. There's no guarantee that you will need surgery or a stoma bag.

P: I'm willing to do anything. I'll stop smoking and I'll eat healthier. Do you think I'll be OK then?

D: It's difficult to say. You are obviously unwell and we need to try getting things back under control. I'll have a word with Dr Thompson. I know things are very tough for you at the moment, especially with the wedding coming up and work. What do you do?

P: I'm an events manager and it's a busy time, you know. Work is good and I enjoy it, but it is really busy at the moment and I need to get it all done.

D: Do you work for yourself or a company?

**Exploring impact upon work/relationship**

P: A company.

D: And do they know what's been going on?

P: Yes, they know. I'm in and out of hospital you see, but they have been really good about it.

D: Well if you need a note to give work then please let me know. I'll also have a word with Dr Thompson and get him to talk to you again.

P: Yeah but please don't tell him about me not taking my medicines.

D: I think it would help if I did tell him as he will need to take that into consideration when deciding what the best treatment may be.

**Avoiding collusion with the patient**

P: Do you think he will be angry?

| Transcript | Skills demonstrated |
|---|---|
| D: No, I don't. I think he will understand that it is very hard for people to take all their medication all the time. You also mentioned that your fiancé would find it very difficult if you did need surgery. If it came to that I would be very glad to talk to him about the surgery and it would also be a good idea to meet the stoma nurse in advance of any possible surgery. | Empathy and showing understanding |
| P: OK, thank you, this has all been very helpful. | |
| D: I know this is very stressful and shocking for you. Is there anything else I can help you with at the moment? | |
| P: No – I think that is everything. | |
| D: Well if you do think of anything do just let me know – you can ask the nurses to bleep me or catch me on the ward rounds. | Organising follow up |

## Patient scenario 15

| Transcript | Skills demonstrated |
|---|---|
| D: Hello Mrs Miah, come in. How are you? | Used patient's name |
| P: Well, I have been better; I just wanted to come in to tell you what's been going on with my pregnancy. | |
| D: OK, please do. | Open question |
| P: I had my 12 week scan; they said the baby had fluid around the neck. So they sent me for more tests, and they did the amniocentesis test. And now they have said that my baby has Down syndrome. They said that is definite. | |
| D: Ah, I am so sorry to hear that. That must have been such a shock for you. | Empathy |
| P: It really was. It has been very stressful. | |
| D: Have you had any thoughts about what to do now? | Exploring ideas |
| P: Well, I'm 17 weeks now. My husband has been saying it's our third baby and just to get a termination. But I've had another scan and I heard the heart beat and I don't want to end it. You know, I'm just going to deal with it as it happens. | |

D: Yes, I can understand that it must be a hard time for you and your husband.

**Empathy**

P: It's also against my religion, you know, it's not something I believe in. I was going to end the pregnancy because of my husband, but I've spoken to lots of people at the hospital and I've decide to keep it and carry on.

D: OK, that's fine. Did you want to talk about the choices or have you already made a firm decision?

P: No, it's been difficult. My husband isn't as strong as me and I don't know how he will deal with it but I've spoken to my mum and I think this is how it was just meant to be and abortion is not something we believe in. So I'm going to carry on with the pregnancy.

D: I know these decisions are always terribly difficult. Did you have any specific questions for me as to what will be happening from now?

**Exploring expectations**

P: Yes, the hospital said I have to have another scan next week. I've just been so tired. I've not been sleeping and I have my other kids – they don't even know. I know there can be a lot wrong with the baby and that we won't know until the baby is born. I am quite worried about it, actually.

D: How have you been coping at home?

**Assessing impact on home/work**

P: Ah, it's not been easy. The kids are picking up on the fact that my husband and I are fighting all the time. And my eldest is 12 and she comes to me and asks why I'm crying and I don't know what to say, to be honest. It's not been good at home and my husband just doesn't want to talk to me right now.

D: So is it still his view that ending the pregnancy would be best?

**Clarifying**

P: Yes, he says I'm selfish, that I haven't thought about the baby and my three girls and how it will impact them. But you know my own mum told me that it's not what we do. We don't have abortions. So it's just something I'm going to have to deal with.

**D:** You mentioned that you have spoken to your mother and have made your decision. Are you happy with the decision you have made or do you feel in any way pressured?

**P:** No, not really, well I guess ... Yes, I do feel pressured but I think I myself couldn't go through with an abortion.

**D:** Have you talked about Down syndrome whilst in the hospital?

**P:** A little but I haven't really taken it all on board, it just feels like it's happening to someone else. I know they will definitely have problems with learning but I don't know.

**D:** You mentioned earlier that you can't tell until the baby is born. To a certain degree that's true but you will have a detailed scan during pregnancy to make sure there are no obvious problems with organs, such as the heart. Have you thought about support groups for parents with Down syndrome children?

Explanation

Support groups

**P:** No I haven't, but that would be really good. I would love to talk to other mums who have been through this. I think that would be a great help, someone that understands what it will be like to go through this.

**D:** I agree and I'll look into that for you and find out if we have any groups locally. You mentioned earlier that you and your husband aren't really speaking – do you think there is anything I could do to help?

Trying to come up with helpful suggestions/ solution

**P:** I don't think so I just wish I hadn't had the amniocentesis test and then we wouldn't have to make the decision. It would have been something we would just have had to deal with.

**D:** Well there are pros and cons to both approaches. I know this is a huge shock for you now but I think it will be best for you to prepare. But you are right, this is a very difficult decision.

**P:** My husband has said that he doesn't want the baby. I'm the one that is carrying it and feeling it move and he has kind of detached himself from it, I think. I don't know how he is going to cope with it all.

**D:** Do you think he will want to come in and talk to someone, a counsellor perhaps?

Offering support for family

**P:** Well he's quite a difficult man so I don't think he will want to talk anyone to be honest.

**D:** It's just that this is a difficult time for you all and I think you're going to need all the support you can get and this is obviously putting a strain on your relationship. Maybe talking to someone might help him.

**P:** Maybe he will be able to speak to you about it. I'll see if I can get him to come in.

**D:** Good, well I'm sure you see his perspective as he does yours and maybe talking will be helpful.

**P:** I think so.

**D:** I am sorry that you are going through this – if there is anything you think that I can do to help, do just let me know.

Empathy

**P:** Thank you. I just wanted to keep you updated on everything.

**D:** Well, come in after you have your second scan and then we can discuss it further.

Organising follow-up

**P:** Thank you.

# Relative scenario 1

| Transcript | Skills demonstrated |
| --- | --- |
| **D:** Good morning Mrs Heath. I'm Dr Dyer, come on in. | Used relative's name |
| **D:** How can I help? | Open question |
| **R:** Well, I've come to speak to you about my husband. | |
| **D:** Yes, of course. | |
| **R:** He's just been diagnosed with coeliac disease and has seen the gastroenterologists but I wanted to talk to you about that. | |
| **D:** OK. Would you be able to tell me what has been happening since he saw them? | Finding out what relative knows and understands already – don't assume |
| **R:** Well, the hospital has been great. One blood test was all it took to diagnose him; he then had a camera test to confirm the diagnosis. He is so much better now he has changed his diet – that is another issue. What I wanted to find out is why on earth this wasn't diagnosed earlier. He was seen here over 6 months ago – it wasn't hard for the hospital doctors after all. | |
| **D:** OK, I can understand why you would be questioning this. Could I spend a moment just recapping what happened when he was first seen | Acknowledging complaint/concern |
| **R:** Well yes, if you can explain why then that would help. | |
| **D:** Looking through the notes it seems that your husband came in to see us with bowel symptoms, he had bloating and abdominal pains. He was investigated with a colonoscopy – this is the test where a small tube is passed through the bowel so that the entire bowel can be examined – this was normal. He also had blood tests that were normal. At this point it was thought that he had a condition called irritable bowel syndrome and ... | |
| **R** [*interrupting*]: I know what was thought but it was wrong. What I want to know is why wasn't he tested for coeliac disease back then. | |

D: You are absolutely right. Coeliac disease was not tested for and it could have been. I don't think it was suspected when your husband was first seen. So I apologise for the delay in the diagnosis. I know it must be very frustrating.

Being open and honest

Empathy

R: It certainly has been – I've been worried sick that he had something going wrong. I thought he probably had cancer but I suppose it's lucky its only coeliac disease.

D: Well yes, in fact I think when your husband was first seen the priority was to rule out cancer – that would be why he had the colonoscopy but I think we need to make every effort to learn from this. I would like to discuss this case with the other doctors in the practice to make sure that similar mistakes don't happen again.

R: I think that is the least that should be done.

D: You said that your husband is much better now – have his symptoms completely resolved?

Reflecting back

R: Yes, when he avoids gluten – but he is getting so bored on the horrible bread he has been prescribed and we can't afford all of the nice products they sell in the supermarket.

D: I can understand that. Would it be OK to move on and talk a bit about the gluten-free diet?

R: Yes – that would be good. I'm a bit lost to be honest. I used to enjoy baking but that is out of the window.

Signposting

D: What have you been told already about the gluten-free diet?

Checking prior knowledge

R: Hardly anything – just what to avoid but it has wrecked our usual diet and my normal cooking.

D: Well, there are so many gluten-free products available on prescription – some patients like some, other patients like others – it is really trial and error. We can also prescribe gluten-free flour to enable you to carry on cooking.

R: Really? I didn't realise that.

**D:** I could leave you some information from Coeliac UK – they do lots of good leaflets, recipes and have lots of good advice. I also think you and your husband would benefit from seeing our dietician because I'm sure you have lots and lots of questions.

Information leaflets and support groups

**R:** That would be really good.

**D:** There is also probably a local support group, which you may find beneficial.

**R:** I'd like that, but I'm not sure about my husband though!

**D:** OK. I know we have talked about a lot so could I just summarise what has been discussed today?

Signposting

**R:** OK.

**D:** You are understandably upset that your husband wasn't diagnosed earlier and I certainly want to look into this in detail, talk to the doctor who saw your husband and make sure that this doesn't happen again. Your husband is much better now he has cut gluten out of his diet but it is restricting your cooking greatly. I think you should try a few more products – and I can leave a script for you, and I will also leave some information leaflets from Coeliac UK as well as referring you to our dietician. Is that OK?

Summarising

**R:** That is right, I'm sorry to complain. I just think other people shouldn't suffer.

**D:** I agree – it's important to learn from these things. Is there anything else I can help you with today?

Acknowledging errors and showing humility

**R:** No, that is it. Thank you.

## Relative scenario 2

| Transcript | Skills demonstrated |
| --- | --- |
| **D:** Hello Mr. Young, come on in. I am Dr Leahy | Used relative's name |
| **D:** How can I help today? | Open question |
| **R:** Well, I'm not really here to talk about me. I'm here to ask your advice about my father. He's one of your patients and I'm really worried about him. | |

**D:** Of course, would you mind telling me a bit more about what you're concerned about?

Open question

**R:** It's nothing specific, I just think he's being quite vague. I don't know, maybe I'm just being silly but he just seems to be getting worse.

**D:** OK, you say he's getting vague. Can you just tell me a bit more about what you have noticed?

Open question to encourage relative to talk

**R:** Yes, well he is quite an intelligent man, but recently he seems quite confused. He has been doing things that aren't quite appropriate like ringing us in the middle of the night.

**D:** I can understand that it is quite stressful for you. Is there anything else that you have noticed that is worrying you?

Empathy and encouragement

**R:** He isn't doing his normal activities; he seems to be going out and about at strange times of the day. My daughter found him walking around town, he didn't know where he was going or what he was doing, and it's getting quite worrying.

**D:** I am sure it is; does he live alone?

**R:** Yes, my mother passed away quite some time ago, so he's been on his own for about 10 years now.

**D:** How do you feel he is coping?

**R:** I think after my mum passed away he was grieving for a long time, but he took care of himself and his house. But for the past few months, when we have met he is getting scruffier, he looks thinner I don't know if he's eating properly. He just doesn't look himself, and I don't think he's looking after himself anymore.

**D:** OK, well it's good that you have come in. This sounds like a very important issue that we need to look into. Do your mind if I ask you a few specific questions?

Signposting

**R:** No, of course not.

**D:** You mention that he's been found wandering outside, have you ever found that he's left the house and left the door open?

Specific questions

**R:** Yes, I think he has done that a few times.

**D:** Has he ever left the gas on at home?

**R:** I'm not aware of that, but he is doing lots of things that seem silly. Like he goes out driving and in the last couple of months he's called me at least three times as he's run out of petrol. This isn't like him, he's usually a switched-on man.

**D:** You mentioned he drives; do you feel that he's safe driving at the moment?

Recognising risk

**R:** Well, how can he be if he's so vague? If he's not thinking about the petrol tank being full is he really paying attention to the roads? It's difficult as I'm very busy and I don't think I have enough time to look after him as much he probably needs.

**D:** I think it's a really good thing that you've come in today. I was just wondering if you have any thoughts as to what may be causing this.

Exploring ICE

**R:** We have a family history of dementia. My grandma had Alzheimer's and I was a teenager at the time so I can't remember much but it does seem like some of these things are similar. I am very worried about that.

**D:** Yes, I can understand that this must be distressing for you. You may well be right, some of the things you are describing, like your father's disorientation and forgetfulness, do sound like early signs of dementia but there are other conditions that cause similar things. Does he drink at all?

Empathy

**R:** He usually has a whisky before bed, and usually at family parties but he's never been a heavy drinker.

**D:** OK, well it's very important that I look into this in more detail. I think it would be best if I could see your father and also organise a few tests. He certainly needs a memory test, and possibly blood tests and a scan of his brain.

Explaining potential outcome for relative

**R:** OK well, that may be a problem, as he doesn't come to the doctors. That's why I've come to see you. You can probably see from his records that he hasn't been in for years.

**D:** Yes, this is often the case in these situations, where the person suffering with the memory problems doesn't want to come in to the doctors.

**R:** How am I meant to bring it up with him?

**D:** It's always going to be difficult, sometimes just being open and saying that you've noticed that he's a little bit forgetful and that the doctor may be able to help may work, but if it's too hard for him to come in then we can certainly visit him at home. It would help if you were there so there is a friendly face for him, so it's not too much of a shock. I am also worried about him continuing to drive, he could be putting himself and others at risk. Do you think you could talk to him to persuade him not to drive?

Problem solving

Advising actions be taken to prevent relative coming to harm

**R:** Yes, I am worried about that as well, I will talk to him. If he says he won't see a doctor, what shall I do?

**D:** We'll cross that bridge when we come to it. If he doesn't want to come in then we can see if he will see me when I visit him at home.

**R:** If you do think he has dementia what happens next?

**D:** The next step would be to organise some blood tests, to make sure there's nothing that could be causing this, and the scan of his brain. We can then take it from there. There are medications that we can use to control it, but at the moment this is all hypothetical and we need to assess your father first.

**R:** I'm just really worried because when my grandma got really unwell she was so distressed and she didn't recognise us. If it has also happened to my father then I suppose it's only time until I also get it.

**D:** I can understand why you are worried but there is no reason to think it will affect you. It is true that there is a very slightly increased chance of being affected if you have a family history of dementia but the chance of not being affected is much higher that the chance of being affected. You mentioned earlier that you are very busy and you think your father needs more help than you can give. How are you coping generally with all of this?

Empathy

Responding to cues

Reassurance

Reflecting back

**R:** Well you know, I just feel really stressed, I worry a lot about my dad and I'm also worried about my own health. Is there anything else I can do to stop myself getting unwell like this?

**D:** I appreciate why you are so concerned, and I am really pleased you have told me about these things but I think there are too many uncertainties at the moment. We don't know that your father has dementia but I would be very willing to talk to you about this in more detail once a firm diagnosis has been made. There are many other conditions that can cause very similar symptoms. He could have an infection, have problems with his thyroid gland or he could be depressed. There are so many things other than dementia, and while we have to rule that out, I don't think it's overly helpful making these suggestions or talking about treatment options. I also really don't think even if he did have dementia that you should be overly worried that you will get it.

Empathy

Explaining differential diagnoses and trying to realistically alleviate some of the relative's concerns

**R:** OK. Thank you, I understand.

**D:** It's very important that we arrange to see your father.

**R:** Yes, that would be good.

**D:** So, to summarise: you and your family have noticed that your father has been getting confused, forgetful and behaving strangely. This may be a sign of dementia but there are other things we need to look into and so I'll meet your father and if possible do a few assessments. Is that OK?

Summarising

**R:** That sounds like a good plan.

**D:** Perhaps we could speak in a few days time and you can let me know if you have persuaded him to come in?

Organising follow-up

**R:** OK, I will do. Thanks.

## Relative scenario 3

| Transcript | Skills demonstrated |
|---|---|
| **D:** Hello Mrs Lucas. I am Dr Benn, come on in. | Used relative's name |
| **R:** Thank you. | |
| **D:** How can I help today? | Open question |
| **R:** I've just come in to speak about my son, Tom. I'm just really worried about him. | |
| **D:** OK, could you tell me more? | Open question |
| **R:** It's not so much his physical health, it's just that he's really changed recently. | |
| **D:** What is it that you have noticed? | Open question |
| **R:** Well, he used to be such a happy-go-lucky boy, a pleasure to get along with. But recently I've been struggling to get him to go to school in the mornings. He tries to stay at home as much as possible. | |
| **D:** It must be quite upsetting for you? | Empathy |
| **R:** Yes, I want him to enjoy school but he keeps saying he has tummy pains all the time and I'm not convinced. | |
| **D:** How long has this been going on for now? | Closed question |
| **R:** Probably a few months. It's probably been a gradual change but for the last few months he definitely hasn't been himself. | |
| **D:** Is there anything else you have noticed which has seemed unusual? | Open exploring question |
| **R:** I don't know if the tummy pains are important or not, he seems to say it most mornings but he doesn't seem to be in pain. I think he is just playing up. | |
| **D:** Yes, abdominal pain in children can often be a sign of stress. Over the past few months have you had any thoughts as to what could be going on that has caused him to change? | Exploring ideas |

R: I've got no idea really; the school keep calling me to go in and to speak about his behaviour. He's never been a naughty child and I can't think of anything specific that could be upsetting him.

D: What sorts of things have been happening at school?

Picking up cues

R: The teachers have told me he has hit other children on two occasions. He's never been a violent boy before and he's always been a pleasure to be with. I don't know if he is the bully or if he's being bullied. I just don't know what's happening.

D: I can understand this must be very stressful for you. Have you spoken to the teachers?

Empathy

R: Yes, I went to seem them when they called me. I asked them if they thought anything was going on and if they thought he was being bullied but they said they haven't noticed anything apart form the change in his behaviour.

D: Have you managed to get any clues as to what could be going on?

Exploring ideas

R: It's very difficult because every time I try and speak to him about it he just says things are fine, and then goes into his room. We are not communicating as we used to.

D: And how are things at home?

R: Things are OK; my marriage broke up last year. My husband and I are separated but I don't know if that can be connected because he seemed OK at the time.

D: So he was OK at the time of your separation but this change in behaviour has started more recently?

Clarifying

R: Yes, things have changed since the break-up. We are both in new relationships and we have both spoken to him about it.

D: OK, could you possibly talk me through the home situation you're in at the moment?

Being 'professionally nosy'

R: I've got a new partner, he doesn't live with us but he and Tom spend a lot of time together. They play together and they get on very well. He's not disruptive or naughty when he's around.

D: OK, and you mentioned that his father is in a new relationship, could you tell me about that please?

R: I don't see much of my ex-husband, but Tom does still sees him a bit, but less often recently.

D: Why is he seeing his father less frequently?

Picking up on cues

R: It used to be every other weekend but he's recently had a new baby with his new wife so it's been a little less at the moment.

D: Do you think that may be affecting Tom at all?

R: Maybe, but because Tom doesn't talk to me about it, I haven't paid it that much attention. It's just so hard to talk to him.

D: It can be incredibly difficult to talk to youngsters like Tom in these kinds of situations, and it is also difficult to pinpoint what is causing the change in his behaviour. It's likely that it's not something he would be able to tell you.

Reassurance

R: Do you think it's some sort of medical issue?

D: Well, it doesn't seem like that, however I can understand why you may think that. I think it's best if I would be able to see Tom myself, try to talk to him and maybe examine him. I think this change you have been noticing is probably related to all of the changes he's gone through in the past year.

R: OK, is there anything that I can be doing better?

D: I really don't think you should be upset, or worry that you should have done anything differently. Marital break ups can be very stressful for children and you just need to provide a supportive and loving environment for Tom. If his behaviour continues to be difficult then we may be able to arrange a counsellor. Before that, though, it may be worth speaking to his father to see if he can see him a bit more, as you mentioned that he hasn't been seeing him much. Maybe he is feeling left out?

Empathy and support

R: Yes, I probably haven't paid that as much attention to that as I should have done. Maybe I should talk to Tom's father about it.

D: It's always difficult to pinpoint what the problem is exactly but it is important to spend as much quality time with Tom as you can.

R: Yes, I suppose I have been quite busy with my own things and work.

D: What is it that you do?

Picking up on cues

R: I work in a bookshop, so the hours are flexible and they coincide with Tom's school. Maybe I have been working too much and I'm probably tired when I pick him up from school and then I see my partner.

D: Yes, it must be very difficult. I think it's good that you have come in to see me today. I know it's difficult to not have an instant solution, but if you could bring Tom in then we can all have a chat together. If its easier for you with work and Tom's school commitments we do have early morning and late evening appointments available

Empathy

R: Thank you – that would be a big help.

D: So perhaps it would be a good idea to speak again privately after I have met Tom.

Organising follow-up

R: That's a good idea. Thank you.

## Relative scenario 4

| Transcript | Skills demonstrated |
|---|---|
| D: Hello Mrs Nicholls, I'm Dr Kumar, one of the doctors on the ward. The ward clerk told me that you wanted a chat? | Used relative's name |
| R: Yes, I just want to complain about how my mother has been looked after on the ward. | |
| D: OK, please tell me what's been happening. | Open question |
| R: My mother, Mrs. Nicholls, has been admitted with a urine infection. Frankly I'm just disgusted by the level of treatment and care she's been getting. | |

**D:** I'm sorry about that. Could you tell me what has been happening?

Maintaining calm approach and exploring issues

**R:** Well, she hasn't been able to maintain any of her dignity, and she's got new pressure sores, which she didn't have in the nursing home and it must be because no one's bothered to turn her around.

**D:** That does sound very distressing.

Empathy

**R:** Yes it's horrible, her skin is obviously fragile. How else would you get pressure sores apart from not being turned around properly?

**D:** You're right; developing pressure sores is something we really try to avoid in patients. I can see why you're upset about this.

Honesty and avoiding 'cover-up'

**R:** Every day I come in and visit her and every time there is something that she isn't happy with. A few times I've seen her she's been totally covered in urine. It's not like she doesn't care or doesn't know what's happening to her. She has asked for a bed pan and no one can be bothered to bring it to her.

**D:** Well, what you're describing sounds very upsetting. It seems as though your mother has not been treated as well as she should have been. Everyone does strive to provide the best care, and sometimes we fall short. It is very good that you have brought this to our attention because it certainly needs to be looked into.

Empathy and explanation

**R:** Obviously my mother is my main concern, but I don't think it's just her. Every time I come and visit I hear the other patients calling out for help. I've gone over and spoken to the other patients and the nurses never come. They just simply don't care.

**D:** OK, I appreciate why you're upset about this. Your mother has obviously had a difficult time here and I certainly need to look into this in more detail to find out what exactly has gone wrong. I will look into why she has developed a new pressure sore and how she's getting on with her treatment. As I said it is really good that you've raised this. I know that it doesn't help your mother, but if there are failings in the nursing care then that really needs to be looked at straightaway so we can improve.

Empathy

Offering to find out more

R: With all respect doctor, I can tell you for a fact that she has been receiving substandard nursing care for a while now. She's not even been fed properly whilst she's here.

D: What have you noticed?

R: One evening I came to visit there was a plate of cold food in her room. This was left on the table on the other side of the room. So it's not as if she wasn't hungry, she just wasn't offered any help to eat.

D: OK, well that is obviously unacceptable and is something that needs to be investigated.

R: You know she came from a nursing home and the standard of care is a hundred times better than this.

D: Have you tried to talk to anyone else about this?

R: I've tried to talk to the nurses but it's very difficult. They just complain that they are too busy, or they are just sat around talking to each other. It's been very hard trying to get someone to talk to. You're the first doctor I've had the opportunity to speak to properly. I just want to know what's going to happen and what you're going to do about this.

D: OK, well thank you for speaking to me about this. I know it's hard to make these sorts of complaints. It is very important that relatives or patients do bring these things to our attention. I think I need to go and speak to the ward sister, examine your mother's pressure sore and work out what treatment she may need. I also plan to check that the urine infection is being treated and she is ready to go back to the nursing home. The next thing is to look into why this has been happening. I will be talking to the ward sister, because a lot of the issues you have raised are to do with the nursing care. The third thing would be for you to think about making a formal complaint. That can be useful for you to do so you can get a proper written explanation. To do that you can speak to the patients' advisory liaisons officers, or PALS, down in the reception of the hospital.

*Summarising plan, acknowledgement of complaint*

*Attempt to move on from relative's anger*

R: Yes, well, I'm not usually someone who makes complaints or makes a big fuss, but this has made me very upset, and I don't want it to happen to anyone else.

**D:** As I say, it is important that we find out when things go wrong. We really do need to look into this and make sure there aren't reasons behind this. I'm not aware of any particular nursing issues on the ward. I would like to thank you for coming in and bringing it to our attention. Can I just ask you a few questions as to how your mother is getting on otherwise?

**R:** Yes, of course.

**D:** How do you feel your mother is getting on with the urine infection?

**R:** She's much better. She's had her treatment for the infection and it's made her a lot better in that she's back to her normal self. She's not so confused any more. It's just that I'm worried that if something like this happens again I won't be able to get her back to the hospital.

**D:** Would it help if I had a word with her and let her know that I am aware of the problems she's had and that we are looking into everything's that's happened to her since she's been here?

**R:** Yes, I think that would be really helpful. I think she would like her chance to explain what's been going on herself.

**D:** OK, I'll certainly do that. I will also take a look at her pressure sores. Would it be helpful if we met in a few days time before she leaves and involve the ward sister as well?

**R:** Well yes, but I don't want my complaint to impact the remainder of my mother's care.

**D:** No, that will certainly not happen.

**R:** OK, well that will be good then.

**D:** I am sorry that you and your mother have been through all this. So if we meet in 2 days time and then we can talk a bit more about what's been happening.

**R:** Thank you.

Signposting

Involving relative in plan

Organising follow-up

# Relative scenario 5

| Transcript | Skills demonstrated |
|---|---|
| **D:** Hello Ms Lewis, I'm Dr Green, the junior doctor on the ward. I understand that you wanted to speak to me. | Used relative's name |
| **R:** I'm James' mum. I just wanted to speak to you about his condition. | |
| **D:** Of course, how can I help? | Open question |
| **R:** Well, James has come in with his asthma again; he was here 6 months ago. I'm very worried about his asthma, do you know why it's getting worse? Do you think it's getting worse? | |
| **D:** Can you tell me a bit more about his asthma? | Open question to find out more information before trying to answer questions directly |
| **R:** He's had it since he was 3 years old, but it's never been a real problem. He came in once when he was 3, when it got quite bad. Then he had to come in 6 months ago, and now we are here again. We are always quite good at controlling it, he takes all his pumps and we manage it well usually. | |
| **D:** OK, did you have any thoughts as to what may be causing this? | Exploring ideas and concerns |
| **R:** I know that I look after his asthma properly, but quite often he stays with his father and I don't know what kind of treatment he gets there. I don't even know whether he is getting his inhalers. | |
| **D:** Have you spoken to James or his father about your concerns? | |
| **R:** Well, James enjoys going to see his father and he doesn't mention anything. I don't really speak to his father anymore. | |
| **D:** How often does he stay with his father? | |
| **R:** Well, we have joint custody so he's with me during the week, and then every second weekend he goes to his father's. | |
| **D:** You mention that you're worried that he isn't having his inhalers – could you tell me a bit more about that? | Reflecting back and clarifying |

R: I can see it, because when he comes back after weekends with his father his breathing is so much worse.

D: You also mentioned that you do not speak to his father.

Reflecting back (demonstrating that you have been listening)

R: We speak when he picks James up but it's a strained relationship and we don't talk properly.

D: OK, does James's father smoke? Or have any pets?

R: Alex never smoked when I was with him, and I don't think he has any pets – James would have told me that but I have noticed that when James come back after a weekend at his Dad's he smells of smoke. I can smell it on his clothes. I don't know, maybe Alex's new girlfriend is smoking but when I ask him about it he says no.

D: Well that would be very important to find out; it is well known that cigarette smoke can make asthma worse.

R: I feel exactly the same doctor but when I ask he just brushes me off, and says no. I don't think he is taking James' asthma seriously.

D: I can understand this must be very stressful for you. Can I just clarify a few details? Would you say that James' current treatment is working most of the time?

Empathy

R: Yes, he has his steroid pump – the brown one that we use and we hardly have to use his blue inhaler.

D: OK, obviously there are these issues with Alex that need to be resolved. Have you any thoughts on how to get more information?

Getting the relative to talk and air their thoughts about possible solutions

R: I think I really need some help with that. I don't want to stop James seeing his father but I don't know how to deal with it if he's not looking after him properly.

D: Yes, it is a difficult situation. Is Alex going to come and see James at any point while he's in hospital?

R: I really doubt it, he doesn't seem to think it's all that serious. Our marriage ended quite badly. It was my entire fault really, so I find it hard to talk about these things with him.

**D:** You mention it ended badly, was it very difficult for you?

*Picking up on cues*

**R:** Yes, we weren't talking to each other for some time; I think our marriage had broken-up a long time ago. But near the end, I am ashamed to say I had an affair. So I feel like I can't complain about Alex as it's my fault.

**D:** Yes I can understand it must be very difficult for you. Does Alex live nearby?

*Empathy*

**R:** Yes, he lives about 10 minutes away.

**D:** OK, I'm just trying to think about what would be the best way to approach this. Obviously you've tried to have a discussion with Alex and it's been difficult. Do you think you would be able to get any further with him?

*Demonstrating your thoughts process to the examiner*

**R:** I don't think I can. I want him to be a part of James life, but I don't think I trust him anymore.

**D:** The other option would be to arrange for Alex to come in and see one of the respiratory nurses, so they can go through everything with him, like using the inhalers properly, and what to do in an emergency. They can also address whether there is any smoking in the house or areas of dust collection.

**R:** How would you arrange that?

**D:** Well I'm not entirely sure to be honest – I would want to discuss this with a colleague who may have dealt with similar situations in the past but I suppose we could contact Alex, on the basis that James has been in twice in a 6-month period with his asthma, and use this as an educational opportunity to prevent any more hospital stays.

*Showing that you would seek help, while still giving suggestions. Verbalising your thoughts*

**R:** What if he says no?

**D:** Well, I haven't come across a situation like this before, so I would have to speak to my consultant to come up with another plan. Just thinking about it now, other options may be to organise health visitors to go round to Alex's house whilst James is there so they can talk through everything.

**R:** Well, I don't want Alex to hate me any more. I don't want our relationship to affect James but I am worried about his health.

**D:** I think you're right. James should come first in this situation. If there is anything that is affecting his asthma. I think that needs to be our primary focus.

Making the patient your primary concern

**R:** I just don't want to be blamed for it.

**D:** I can understand that, I don't think there is any blame here; it purely needs to be about improving James' asthma, to make sure he doesn't come in to the hospital again.

**R:** So you'll speak to Alex?

**D:** Yes I'll have a chat to my consultant and the respiratory nurse, to come up with a plan to talk to Alex. Then maybe it would be good for us to meet up after I've spoken to my team. Did you have anything else that you were worried about?

Organising follow up

**R:** No, I think that's all, thanks.

**D:** OK, thank you for speaking to me. I think you have raised very important issues.

## Relative scenario 6

| Transcript | Skills demonstrated |
|---|---|
| **D:** Hello Mrs Brown, I am Dr Graham. Come on in. How can I help today? | Used relative's name<br>Open question |
| **R:** I just want to know if you've looked at my father's notes and know what's been happening to him? | |
| **D:** Yes, I've read the summary I have here. I am very sorry to learn of your father's diagnosis, this must be a very difficult time for you all. | Empathy |
| **R:** Obviously we are all quite upset about this. | |
| **D:** I'm sure. Would you mind telling me a bit about what has happened? | Open question to explore relative's understanding of events |

R: Well, he's had this cough for a long time but then he started to cough up blood and I took him straight to A&E. He was admitted to the ward and then they diagnosed him with cancer. I just can't believe it, I really can't.

D: It must have come as a huge shock to you all.

*Empathy by acknowledging emotion/ stress*

R: Absolutely, I'm just amazed that this wasn't picked up earlier. He came here a few months ago about his cough. I know he wasn't coughing up blood then but he had the cough and you arranged some tests. But no one even mentioned that cancer was a possible diagnosis.

D: I understand why you are upset at this diagnosis and concerned that it could have been made earlier. Would it be helpful if I went through what happened when he was seen a few months ago?

*Demonstrating you have understood relative frustrations and signposting*

R: Yes, I guess that would be helpful.

D: I am sure you are aware that your father has been a lifelong heavy smoker and has had a cough for many months. During the course of investigations for his cough, we examined him, took a history from him and there wasn't anything that suggested that he had lung cancer. However we did perform a chest X-ray just to make sure there wasn't anything there, like a cancer. Your father's X-ray was normal – there was nothing there to suggest cancer.

*Clear explanation*

R: So was cancer suspected when he was seen a few months ago then?

D: Well yes, whenever someone has a chronic cough we do think about lung cancer and try to rule this out, although I must say most people who present with lung cancer do not present with a cough like your father's. The suspected diagnosis at the time was COPD or emphysema, have you heard of that before?

R: Yes, isn't that the smoker's disease?

D: That is exactly right. The plan was for your father to have a test where he breathes into a machine to make a firm diagnosis.

R: Why hasn't he been seen since then? I had to take him to A&E to get this diagnosis?

**D:** I don't know the full situation here, but from what I can see here he was advised to go and see the nurse for smoking cessation and to book in for the lung function test. But it doesn't look like it has been done.

**R:** So you don't think this could have been caught earlier?

**D:** It's very difficult to say. He did have an X-ray that was reported to be normal. What I can do is to get the hospital to look at the X-ray again to make sure that there isn't anything that may have been missed. If there wasn't, then no, I don't think it realistically could have been diagnosed any earlier.

Acknowledging uncertainty

**R:** I guess that makes sense, obviously we are very worried as to what's going to happen to him now.

**D:** I can understand that. The other thing to say is that even if it had been diagnosed earlier I don't think it would have necessarily altered the treatment plan or the outcome.

**R:** OK, but we don't even know what his treatment is going to be. I know they said they can't operate. I think they will be doing chemotherapy or radiotherapy. I'm just very worried that it will make him very unwell.

**D:** Yes, usually with lung cancer, surgery isn't always an option. Most patients tend to have some form of radiotherapy or chemotherapy. Would you like me to discuss some of the things that will be happening to your father from now on?

Signposting change of direction and focus

**R:** Yes please, because I just don't know if he's able to cope with the treatment. Will he be able to stay at home?

**D:** Could you tell me a bit more about the situation at your father's home?

Getting more information before offering advice/ explanation

**R:** He lives at home with my mother; she isn't too well herself at the moment. She suffers quite badly from rheumatoid arthritis. I end up caring for her quite a lot as it is, and so having to look after my father as well is going to be quite hard.

**D:** Yes, I can see how this must be very hard for you.

Empathy

**R:** I have my own life and my own kids, and now having to look after both my parents, it's obviously very stressful.

**D:** Certainly, we need to make sure that your parents are well enough supported at home and so the pressure isn't on you. Anything you do to help would be in addition to the basic care that he would already be getting.

**R:** So I can get some help?

**D:** Absolutely, have you ever spoken to your parents about getting help at home or have they ever been assessed for that?

Exploring ideas

**R:** Not really as my father has always been well enough to look after everything.

**D:** OK, do you have any thoughts as to what they might need?

**R:** I certainly want them to stay at home, but I know I won't be able to spend a lot of time at their home every day.

**D:** No, of course. We could arrange for a social worker to come round and discuss with them what help they would need. I suppose if your father becomes more unwell with the treatment, we could get carers to come in and help with the shopping and cleaning. They could also get help with getting ready in the morning and other such things, should the need arise.

**R:** Yes, I've been doing all of it for my mother since my father has been unwell, but I'm not sure I can cope with both of them.

**D:** Absolutely and you shouldn't have to. I need to get more information from the hospital as to what the treatment plan is for your father. Did anyone at the hospital go through it with you?

**R:** Yes they did but to be honest with you, I didn't take much of it in. I know they are planning to see my father again next week.

**D:** Would it be helpful to meet after that appointment and so we can discuss what will be happening? It may help if you bring your father in also.

Organising follow-up

R: Yes, I think that will be a good idea.

D: I know you were worried if this could have been picked up earlier, so I will speak to the radiology department and get back to you when we meet again. I know you will have lots of questions over the next few weeks. If you do need to speak to me before we meet, then just give me a call. If your father wants to come in to speak with me I am more than happy to see him too.

| Reflecting back to earlier concerns |
| --- |

R: OK, thank you.

## Relative scenario 7

| Transcript | Skills demonstrated |
| --- | --- |
| D: Hello Mr Potter, I'm Dr Murphy. The nurse mentioned that you wanted to speak to me. How can I help? | Used relative's name<br>Open question |
| R: Well, I just wanted to speak about my mother. Obviously you know she's been in hospital with a broken hip and she's been quite unwell whilst she's been here, but I've spoken to the nurse who thinks she is ready to go home. I just wanted to talk to you about it because I'm very worried. | |
| D: Yes, well it's a very good idea to talk about this. Could you tell me about your concerns? | Open question |
| R: Well even before the accident I don't think she was coping at home. She seems even weaker since she's been in hospital. | |
| D: OK, so you mentioned that even before she came to hospital she wasn't coping. What sorts of things were going wrong? | Open exploring question |
| R: Well, a year ago she was a very sociable lady. She was getting out of the house, visiting friends. She was looking after herself properly, but more recently she is just neglecting herself a lot more. She stays at home, she doesn't go out, and she doesn't see people. She isn't coping at all. | |
| D: You say that she is neglecting herself. What sorts of things have you noticed? | Open question to get all the information |

**R:** Well, when I've gone to visit the house is in a mess. There is clutter everywhere and that is not like her – she used to be proud of her house. She isn't dressing properly or doing her hair. She just isn't taking care of herself in that way anymore.

**D:** Do you have any thoughts as to what may be causing the change in her ability to look after herself?

Exploring ideas

**R:** I don't think she is losing her marbles or anything. I mean we can still have conversations like we used to and she is as sharp as ever. It seems like she is getting weaker and weaker and has no energy or drive to do these things anymore.

**D:** OK, do you mind if I ask a few specific questions?

Signposting

**R:** Go ahead.

**D:** How do you feel her mood is generally?

Specific questions looking into depression and home situation

**R:** She always seems pleased to see us, but I don't think she is going out and about enough to be living life to the full. She does seem a bit low.

**D:** Can you tell me a few things about where she lives and who with?

**R:** She still lives in our family home, where she used to live with my father. He died quite suddenly a few years ago. So she lives in the big house by herself.

**D:** I see. Does she have downstairs toilet?

Appropriate closed questions

**R:** Yes she does, but the proper bathroom is upstairs.

**D:** Has she been managing to get upstairs?

**R:** I think so, but when we visit she does move very slowly. Obviously I'm not there all the time so I can't see what she does all the time.

**D:** It must be stressful and upsetting for you seeing her like this.

Empathy

**R:** Yes, I haven't been happy with this situation for a while now.

**D:** Where do you live?

**R:** I live down in Somerset with my wife and children. My kids are in school there and they are quite settled. So it has been quite difficult with my mother living all the way up here in London.

**D:** Yes, I can see how it must be quite difficult. Have you got any other relatives that could check in on your mother?

Problem solving

**R:** Well, she has a few friends that live near here. I have a sister but she lives in New Zealand. I speak to her regularly but she obviously can't come and visit.

**D:** I understand that you have concerns about her going home. Have you got anything in mind about what should happen?

Exploring ideas and expectations

**R:** I would ideally like her to be closer to us but we don't have the room or the time for her to live with us. I have looked into a residential home near Somerset, which would be ideal.

**D:** Have you talked to your mother about this?

Establishing patient's views

**R:** Yes, I've tried to bring it up on a few occasions but she is very stubborn. She doesn't want to leave her home.

**D:** Yes, these are always very difficult situations for all involved.

**R:** I mean what can we do?

**D:** It's always very tricky, if someone has the ability to make their own decisions, which it sounds like your mother does, then really we need to go along with her wishes. Obviously we need to make sure that she is as safe as possible at home, and that she is able to cope. However, at the end of the day, even if patients make decisions that we may think are not the right ones, we have to give them the right to make their own decisions.

Explaining capacity

**R:** But what do we do to make sure that she is safe?

**D:** OK, there are various things that I think will be important for you talk to your mother about. If she doesn't want to go to a residential home, then maybe she would consider letting carers into her home to check in on her. There are services such as shopping, cleaning and a community alarm. She could wear this alarm, which is basically a small button on a necklace, which raises help when pressed, in case she has another fall and needs help. How would you feel about that?

*Explaining options*

*Conceptual thinking and problem solving*

**R:** Well, they all sound like good ideas; I just don't want her to be discharged before anybody has really thought about these issues.

**D:** Yes, thank you for raising them. All of our patients are assessed before they are discharged. There is a team of people involved: doctors, physiotherapists, nurses, social workers and the occupational therapist. We do a total assessment to see if the patient will be able to cope at home. We certainly need to have a discussion and sometimes we hold a discharge planning meeting which involves the patient and their family. Would you like me to arrange that?

**R:** Yes, I just don't want her to go home without having any help set up.

**D:** It's difficult. I haven't spoken to your mother yet about what she would like to happen. Would it be helpful if I went to speak to her with the social worker? We could then organise a discharge meeting. I would also like to speak to her because some of the things you have mentioned suggest that she may be depressed. This is very common in the elderly, especially in her situation.

*Reflecting back – offering to speak to patient and exploring possible diagnosis of depression*

**R:** Yes, I had wondered whether that might be the case. I think if you expressed some of the concerns that I have she may listen.

**D:** OK, I will certainly do that. You mention that you are living in Somerset. Will you be here for a few more days or should we speak by phone?

*Organising follow-up*

**R:** If we set a date then I can make arrangements. Thank you.

# Relative scenario 8

| Transcript | Skills demonstrated |
|---|---|
| **D:** Good afternoon Mrs Martin, I am Dr Frost. I was told you wanted to speak to me. How can I help? | Used relative's name |
| **R:** Thank you very much for looking after my son Tom. I just wanted to have a chat about what happened that night. | |
| **D:** OK, that's fine, what did you want to talk about? | Open question |
| **R:** Well he took some drugs that night. This was a real shock to me and I've briefly spoken to him about it. He has apologised about it and I think this has given him a big scare. My main issue is that I don't want this to go on his medical record. | |
| **D:** This must have been a great shock for you and your family. You said that you don't want it on his record, why is it that you want it to be taken off? | Empathy<br>Open question to understand the issue |
| **R:** He's only 16 and it's not good for him in general but it's mainly because he has always wanted to join the Army, and I'm petrified that it would ruin his chances if they would ever find out. | |
| **D:** OK, do you think that Tom's drug use would affect his entry into the Army? | Clarifying |
| **R:** Yes, I think they would deny his application. I know they are strict and they look to see if people are fit and healthy. | |
| **D:** Thank you for telling me all about this. I think at this point it would be helpful to talk about what happens to medical records. The records of Tom's consultation are very important and are made in the patient's best interest. They cannot be edited unless it is factually incorrect, for example if somebody had written in the wrong notes by mistake. The information can't be removed either even if they are incorrect; they would just be crossed through and amended. [*pause*] I know that must be upsetting because you are obviously very keen for it to not be on his records. I'm not entirely sure what the Army policy is on this sort of thing. Have you looked into this? | Clear explanation<br><br><br><br><br><br>Empathy |

R: Well, a friend of mine's son was told that he couldn't join because they looked at his notes and saw that he had really bad asthma. I'm just worried that they will look at Tom's record's and say he can't join because of this one episode of drug taking.

D: I think that's a very important point to raise. The Army have very strict policies on health requirements. Severe asthma is something that could affect someone's fitness. I don't know specifically about their rules, but the Army is known for turning people's lives around and they will be aware that a lot of people make mistakes when they are younger. I don't think they would have managed to help so many people if they had very strict requirements.

R: So you think it wouldn't necessarily stop him from joining?

D: I wouldn't have thought so but I don't have a great deal of experience dealing with such issues. I think that it is important to clarify that Tom would need to consent to any medical information being given to the Army. I don't know what information the Army request, or what they would do if Tom did not consent for them to receive his medical report. I would need to look into this further.

Expressing view but being honest about lack of firm knowledge

R: OK, I suppose that is something. I just really wish this hadn't happened and I don't want him to be rejected for this silly mistake. I don't think he could handle it and I'm sure that if he realised that he could still join the Army, he would never touch drugs again.

D: You said that you had briefly spoken to Tom. What did you discuss?

R: Yes, we did speak but I was very angry when this first happened. I know he drinks but most teenagers do but I had never thought he would be into drugs. I've managed to calm down now and want to speak to him about it properly.

D: Yes, it must have been a big shock for you. How is Tom getting on generally?

R: He is doing well. He is not academic but he tries hard and gets good reports. He is very sociable and has lots of friends. I've always liked his friends but maybe he is in with the wrong crowd.

**D:** What makes you think that?

Picking up cues

**R:** I just wonder who he got these drugs from. I know it was a massive party and there were lots of people I don't know there.

**D:** Maybe when you get home Tom may speak to you about it a bit more.

**R:** I hope so. I am just so worried about this being on his record. I might also just ask my GP what is likely to happen – they may have dealt with this sort of thing before.

**D:** Yes, that sounds a very good idea. We will send a discharge summary to the GP; I'm not entirely sure what happens to the information at the GP practice. I may have a chat with Tom just to reiterate the importance of staying away from drugs and you may find information on drugs helpful – there are lots of websites designed for young people like Tom that you may also find useful – one that comes to mind is 'Talk to Frank'.

**R:** Yes, I think I have heard about that one. Thank you.

## Relative scenario 9

| Transcript | Skills demonstrated |
| --- | --- |
| **D:** Hello Mr Jones. I am Dr Bartley. Come on in. | Used relative's name |
| **D:** How can I help? | Open question |
| **R:** I think you've been looking after my mum, is that right? | |
| **D:** Yes that is right, I have been. | |
| **R:** Yes, thanks. I think she's doing a lot better now, but the thought of her going back to that nursing home is just unbearable. | |
| **D:** Can you tell me a bit more about that? | Open question |
| **R:** I'm kicking myself, you know. I think things have been going on for ages. Since she's been in hospital she looks better and she looks happier. | |
| **D:** I'm glad that you are happy with the care she has received here but can you tell me a bit more about why you don't want her to return to the nursing home? | |

**R:** The staff don't care at all. I have no idea why they are nurses. The stuff I have seen has just horrified me. She really can't go back there, even if it's just for a few weeks.

**D:** Could you tell me what you have seen?

Picking up on cues

**R:** I know it must be hard, they have a lot of patients, but I've seen confused patients who just want to have a wander round get thrust back into their seats by these 'nurses'. I've seen patients who have tried to eat but they need help and their food is just left on the side. There have been times where my wife and I have helped out. I also kept telling them that my mum had this really nasty chesty cough and seemed breathless. The nurses just kept saying that she was fine and eventually she has ended up in hospital. If they had just listened and cared from the beginning then it wouldn't have got this bad.

**D:** I can understand why this is so distressing for you and it sounds as though you have seen some really unacceptable things. Do you mind if I ask you a few specific questions to clarify a few things?

Empathy and acknowledging seriousness of issues early. Signposting

**R:** No, not at all.

**D:** How long has she been there for?

**R:** For nearly a year I think. Far too long, I feel dreadful about it.

**D:** Have you always been unhappy with the care there?

**R:** It's one of things that just dawns on you. I think back on everything I've seen and I wonder how I've let this go on for so long.

**D:** Have you spoken to your mum about how she feels about being there?

Trying to establish patient's views

**R:** I keep asking her but she thinks she's a burden on us. We don't live close by so she just says she's OK but I know she's not.

**D:** Yes, I can see how distressing this must be for you. You mentioned earlier that you don't live close by.

Reflecting back what the relative had said previously

**R:** I live in Manchester, and my mum's nursing home is in London. So it was difficult because we moved up there about 18 months ago for my job. At the time we talked about taking her up with us, either for her to move in with us or into a nursing home there. We spoke to her GP, who is really excellent and he thought it would have been too disruptive for her, she has friends here and she goes to the day centre and everything. I think with hindsight it would have been better to take her with us at the time.

**D:** OK, is that something that is on your mind at the moment, are you hoping to move her?

**R:** I think with the experience I have had with this nursing home I just can't bear for her to be there anymore.

**D:** Have you tried to speak to someone at the home?

**R:** In the past yes, I have tried, I mentioned about how the patients needed help eating and they just say 'yeah, yeah, yeah,' and don't actually do anything. To be honest I can't be bothered, I don't see that it's going to change, it's not just one nurse it's the whole place.

**D:** You mentioned that your wife had noticed this too. Does your mother have any other visitors?

**R:** My children come down when we go; they find it difficult to see their nanny in that place.

**D:** You said that she had friends and went to the day centre.

**R:** Yeah well, most of them are too ill to visit, or have passed on. She has a few people in the nursing home she gets on with but I wouldn't call them her friends.

**D:** OK, would you mind if I just summarised everything to make sure I haven't missed anything out?

**R:** Yeah sure.

**D:** So I understand that you are quite anxious that your mother is going to be discharged, and going back to the nursing home because you have witnessed very poor care from the nursing staff. You are hoping to maybe move her closer to you, but nothing has been put in place at the moment. You've spoken to your mother but she doesn't seem to complain about anything, as she doesn't want to burden you.

Summarising

**R:** Yes, that's about it.

**D:** Have you had any other thoughts about what we can do to help?

Exploring expectations

**R:** I just want her to stay here to be honest until I can arrange something else.

**D:** These are very serious things that you have noticed and I think the care at the nursing home will probably need to be formally investigated. I will definitely have to speak to my team about this. [*Pause.*]

**D:** I'm not sure that it is a good idea to keep patients on an acute hospital ward while you look for somewhere for her to go. There is always the risk of exposure to other infections and of course the beds are always in high demand. I do understand your concerns though and want to reassure you that we won't discharge your mother without proper thought. I think the best thing for me to do would be to speak to the social workers and the discharge team who can look into this for you and discuss this further.

Clear honest explanation

Empathy

**R:** Yes, I think that would be best because I do not want her to go back there.

**D:** Yes, of course. I'm not too sure how it works entirely but I know that we have rehab centres where she can go in the interim. Have you thought about making a formal complaint against the nursing home yourself?

Verbalising thoughts

**R:** I haven't really, do you think I should?

**D:** Well, you have noticed some very worrying things that need to be investigated.

Acknowledging seriousness of issues again

**R:** Yes, I think I probably should, just for the sake of the other patients.

**D:** OK, well I will arrange the meeting with the discharge team for you and they can talk through your options. I will also speak to the social worker about the way that the care at the nursing home can be looked into. How does that sound?

Explaining ongoing plan and seeking agreement

**R:** Thank you, that sounds good.

D: OK, well it is really good that you have brought these issues to my attention.

R: Thank you

## Relative scenario 10

| Transcript | Skills demonstrated |
|---|---|
| D: Hello Ms West, I am Dr Fitzpatrick. Come on in. How can I help today? | Used relative's name<br>Open question |
| R: Hi, I just wanted to chat to you about my mum. I'm not sure if you know her? | |
| D: No, I've not met your mother yet, but I've read through her notes. | |
| R: OK, I'm just a bit worried about her. I just wanted to chat about what's been going on. | |
| D: Yes of course, tell me what's been going on. | Open question |
| R: She's 94 and she's doing quite well but I'm just worried about how she will cope. She has quite arthritic knees and she needs a lot of help, especially with the stairs. I help her out mostly and I think I'm taking the brunt of this. She's quite stubborn and she doesn't want to have any other help. | |
| D: You mention that you are taking the brunt of it. What are you doing exactly to help? | Reflecting back and clarifying details |
| R: I don't live with her which is part of the problem. I live locally so I go round in the morning, get her up, washed and dressed and ready for the day and then I go back in the evening and make her dinner and help her to bed. | |
| D: That does sound like a lot of work and it sounds like you are her full-time carer. | |
| R: Yes, I guess I am, as well as having my own job! | |
| D: Have you ever thought about getting some professional help? | |

R: I would love some help. You know, a lot of my friends have parents who are the same age as my mum and they all think I'm mad doing this all alone but as I said my mum is very stubborn and she won't accept help from anyone else.

D: You mention that she doesn't want any help; do you have any thoughts as to why?

Exploring ideas

R: Yes, my father passed away a few years ago, and he required carers. They basically came when they wanted; they would come at 5 pm to put him to bed and he wasn't really looked after properly. His last few months weren't great. So she has a very poor view of carers and doesn't want to be treated like that.

D: Yes, that is understandable. Some of my patients have described similar problems with carers in the past, but the provision of care has now changed, and there is more choice as to who provides the care.

R: That's the other thing, we didn't know who the carer was with my father, and they were different every day. She won't open the door to anyone that she doesn't recognise, so it would be hard.

D: Do you think she realises the strain it is putting on you?

Empathy and appreciating stress of being a carer

R: I try not to show it to her, I would feel guilty for making her feel like a burden. At the end of the day I am her daughter and I am willing to help. I know that she does appreciate me but I don't think she knows how much it's affecting me.

D: How is it affecting you, if you don't mind me asking?

R: I think it was fine up until recently. I was working very regular hours so I was managing her care around work. But it's all a bit of a mess at the moment as I have to do other things as well.

D: What is it that you do?

Exploring psychosocial factors

R: I'm a librarian.

D: That must be a lot of work in addition to all of your caring responsibilities. How is it going?

R: Good, I love it. I've been there for years and as I said I work regular hours, from 10 am to 4 pm, so it was OK. But recently things have been chaotic.

D: What's been going on that has changed things?

R: Well I've had a few health problems of my own; obviously I haven't told my mother this. She would just be so worried. I've had some bleeding and I had to be referred. I've been diagnosed with cancer of the womb. Luckily they don't think it has spread and I have to have surgery in the next couple of weeks.

Picking up cue

D: I am very sorry to hear that. This must be very hard for you. Obviously, with having surgery and the recovery time you will need after this, I think it will be unwise for you to be caring for your mother during that time. What are your thoughts about that?

Empathy

R: Yes, they told me that I won't be able to do heavy lifting for at least 6 weeks.

D: I think you should try to take this as an opportunity to change the way your mother is cared for.

R: Yes well, I suppose that's why I have come in today.

D: Have you tried talking to her about this?

R: I don't know how to begin really and I don't want to worry her.

D: Well I think your mother will obviously know that you will be going in for surgery because you won't be there for a few days and due to the fact that you will not be able to do things afterwards. It may be wise to have an open conversation about things. I appreciate that you don't want to burden her but your health needs to take priority here. Maybe you don't need to mention the severity of the condition if you don't want to worry her. There are options for her to go to a respite home, but if she doesn't want to leave, then she needs to consider carers.

Explanation

Demonstrating active listening by reflecting upon previously expressed concerns

**R:** Yes, I think I've known this is the only way for a long time. I just don't want her to feel guilty for being a burden on me.

**D:** I am sure that she will understand that you need to look after yourself too. There are clear reasons for you to involve carers. I can put you in touch with a social worker and see what they have to offer. You can all discuss the issues you had with your father's carers so you can see what will work best for everyone.

Conceptual thinking

**R:** Yes, that will be good.

**D:** So I will leave the details for the social worker at reception for you. If you have any problems just contact me. I think it would also be helpful if I visited your mother when you're in hospital to see if she's OK – that may give you a bit of peace of mind as well.

**R:** That would be great; you will be able to see how unsuitable the house is.

**D:** What are the problems there?

Picking up cue (last minute)

**R:** Well, it's mainly the stairs, getting her up and down is hard. It's just not ideal but luckily we have a toilet downstairs.

**D:** We can ask the occupational therapist to speak to you too as they may be able to organise a stair lift to be put in.

**R:** Yes, that would be great. OK, I'll speak to them and see what they say. Thanks.

# Relative scenario 11

| Transcript | Skills demonstrated |
| --- | --- |
| **D:** Hi there Mrs Jameson, come through. I am Mark Fraser. How can I help you? | Used relative's name |
| **R:** I wanted to talk about Mike, my husband who is a patient here. I'm just so worried about him. I really hate to be coming here and talking about him but I just don't know what else to do. | |
| **D:** Could you tell me some more? | Open question |
| **R:** Well, he has a problem drinking. He doesn't really understand that it's become such a big problem but I can assure you it really has! It's now starting to affect me and I just don't know what I'm supposed to do. | |
| **D:** I'm glad you've come here today. Do you want to start from the beginning? | Open question |
| **R:** Well, Mike and I have always enjoyed a couple of glasses of wine in the evenings on most nights, which I know is probably too much anyway but he's having a lot more now. Lately, I just don't really think I know him anymore. As you probably know from seeing him here, he's a consultant anaesthetist down the road and things have just been awful for him over the last 7 months. He's changed. | |
| **D:** What sort of changes have you noticed? | Open question |
| **R:** He doesn't want to go out or see his friends. He's not that interested in our girls anymore. It's so worrying and I don't know how to help him … | |
| **D:** That sounds very stressful. Do you have any idea why he may have changed like this? | Exploring ideas |
| **R:** There was an incident at work just before he started drinking more. At the time there was a big investigation going on because a young healthy patient having a routine procedure died on the operating table, and although his name's been cleared now, I know he still thinks about it and feels somewhat responsible for the whole thing. | |
| **D:** Gosh, that sounds terrible. | Empathy |

**R:** Yes it was. It was a really terrible time for the whole family and poor Mike. And since then things have just taken a turn for the worst for us all.

**D:** Has you spoken to him about all of this?

**R:** I tried. Initially the investigation was all he could ever talk about. He has always moaned about pressure at work. Now he just comes home late from work and barely says anything.

**D:** You also expressed concerns that he is drinking too much.

Reflecting back

**R:** Yes. I think he is. He gets home and opens a bottle of wine, then he has some whisky. Sometimes he gets up in the middle of the night and wanders around the house. There was a time I found him in the living room at 3 in the morning drinking even more whisky. He said it was to help him sleep. I am so worried, I have thrown so much alcohol away.

**D:** Do you ever worry that he may not be able to perform at work, especially considering his drinking?

Ensuring safety

**R:** No, not at all. I mean he has been drinking in the night a few times but he has never been drunk going to work and I think if anything he's probably even more careful after everything that happened with that patient.

**D:** And you mentioned your girls earlier. How old are they and are they affected in anyway?

Reflecting back and picking up cues

**R:** They are 12 and 10. They adore their dad and have been asking why he doesn't talk much. I keep saying he's fine but I'm sure they can sense it.

**D:** Have you ever felt that you are worried about Mike looking after them with the way he is at the moment?

Ensuring no child protection issues

**R:** No, not really. I've always been responsible for the kids so there is rarely a time when he has to look after them but I'm not worried. My hours are a lot more manageable than his so that's just how it's been.

**D:** OK. Do you know if Mike has seen anyone for any help or would want to have help?

R: No way. He is very stubborn and with the way he is I can't imagine he would go to anyone for help. I wish he would. I just want someone to help him. Is it possible for you to check if he's been here at all?

D: No, I'm afraid I couldn't do that as that would be breaching his confidentiality. I'm really sorry about that.

Confidentiality

R: Of course. I totally understand.

D: This all seems pretty awful for your whole family. How is this affecting you?

Empathy

R: I'm pretty tough but I must say I am stressed. I work part time at the moment but even then I can't really concentrate there. I am barely sleeping because I want to keep an eye on Mike since I found him drinking at night. I also just miss him. He's not the person I married. We barely speak, let alone have any fun or go out.

D: Have you confided in anyone else?

R: I have told one of the other physios I work with and she's been amazing. I haven't told anyone else though. Our friends keep asking if everything's OK as I keep making excuses whenever we are invited out.

D: OK. Would you mind if I just summarised back to you what you've told me so I can make sure I haven't missed anything? You have been worried about your husband, who is a consultant anaesthetist, for the last 6 months. It seems he has changed following an incident at work and has gone from being quite active and friendly to somewhat reclusive and his behaviour has changed towards you and your children. He has been drinking much more than he used to and he hasn't really accepted there may be a problem.

Summarising

R: Yes, that seems like it really.

D: Have you any thoughts about how you want to handle this?

Exploring thoughts/ expectations

R: Well I think I may need to just have a few weeks at home so I may take some time off work to think things through. I'm so tired I need to make sure I stay strong for the kids. I've thought about asking one of his friends at work if things are OK and seeing if someone can talk to him. I also wanted to try and get him here but I don't know how I could do that.

D: That all seems very reasonable. I agree that you definitely do need to look after yourself and if you do need some time off work I would be more than happy to give you a note for your employer, if they need it.

R: That would be great.

D: Do you think you may be able to persuade Mike to come in, possibly even with you?

R: I can try and ask him.

D: I know time is short today but it seems there is a lot more we should discuss with regards to your wellbeing and the situation in general. Do you think you would be able to come back next week to see me? Maybe a double appointment would be better.

Time management
Organising follow-up and recognising the need to address further issues

R: That would be great. In the meantime I can try and convince Mike to come with me.

D: Yes, that would be ideal if you could bring him. If he is not keen you could try and convince him to speak to someone in occupational health as well. Is there anything else you wanted to mention today?

R: No, that's fine. I feel much better already for just talking to someone about it.

D: I hope you're OK and I'll see you next week. If there is anything else you want to talk to me about before then please leave a message for me and I can call you back.

R: Thanks so much Dr Fraser. See you next week.

## Relative scenario 12

| Transcript | Skills demonstrated |
| --- | --- |
| D: Hello Mrs Johnson. Come through. My name's Dr Patel. How can I help? | Used relative's name |
| R: Hi Dr Patel, I wanted to speak to you about my son, Paul. | |
| D: Certainly, how can I help? | Open question |

**R:** Well basically I want an epinephrine injectable pen for him.

**D:** OK, could you tell me a bit more about this?

Open question

**R:** His cousin has a severe allergy to bees and almost died of a reaction last week. My sister told me he now has to keep an injectable pen with him at all times and it may be worth keeping one for Paul too.

**D:** I see, I'm sorry to hear about that. How is your nephew doing now?

Empathy

**R:** He's fine now, thank goodness. He was admitted for 2 days though and it was a real scare to everyone.

**D:** I can imagine. Has Paul ever had an allergic reaction before or been stung by a bee?

**R:** No he hasn't. I think he has been stung before but I know allergies can start at any time.

**D:** OK. We can definitely have a chat about that and I can completely understand why you're worried. Can I just ask how Paul's general health is?

Ensuring all facts established before making a plan

**R:** He's fine. Really well actually.

**D:** I'm glad to here that. Do you think we could talk a little bit about what happened to your nephew and the need for injectable pens?

Signposting

**R:** Yes, that's fine.

**D:** It sounds like your nephew, as you said, had an allergic reaction which was severe and that is why he has to carry an epinephrine pen in case he were to be stung again. It is extremely unlikely that your son would have the same reaction as this is quite rare. I can imagine that this is still very worrying for you but usually we only prescribe epinephrine pens for people who have a history of severe allergy.

**R:** So what you're saying is you have to wait for something life-threatening to happen. Is this a cost-saving measure?

D: Well, no. If there was a history of allergy or someone was felt to be at risk then we would consider it but the problem is that the medication in an epinephrine pen is not without its own risks if used inappropriately. It would also be significant burden for Paul – he would have to always carry it with him and we would not want to make him do that unless absolutely necessary.

*Explanation of reasons*

R: OK. So you can't give it to me. Well, what if you test him and see if he is allergic to bees?

D: We could do that, but it is not really as common as you think, but if you are extremely concerned it is of course something we could consider. I understand that this must have been a shock for you but you do seem extremely worried about Paul. I am just wondering whether anything else has happened that could be worrying you?

*Responding to anxiety – openly acknowledging what you are picking up to find out why*

R: My husband thinks I am a panicking mother and that there is nothing to worry about, but Paul is my only child and I worry. Paul had a brother, Jack, who died.

D: I'm so, so sorry to hear that. I can understand why you would feel as you do. It is a natural reaction. Do you mind me asking what happened?

*Empathy*

R: That's OK. It was 7 years ago now. He was 3 months old and died of cot death …

D: I'm sorry to hear that. Are you OK? [*Pause.*] I'm sorry if I've upset you

*Use of silence*

R: That's OK. I haven't really talked about this for ages. It's OK …

D: Would you like to take a moment?

*Empathy*

R: No, it's OK.

D: Well I can totally understand why you're so worried about Paul, having had such a shock before. You mentioned you haven't really spoken about it for a while. Is this something you feel you might still need some support with?

*Picking up on cues*

**R:** No, really. I'm OK. Thanks though.

**D:** How are things at home?

**R:** OK. My husband is great and we've come to terms with things now.

**D:** That's good. How do you feel about Paul not having an Epipen?

Clarifying thoughts and agreement with management plan

**R:** I would really appreciate it if you could get him tested as I do understand you can't give us this pen but I think it would give me some peace of mind.

**D:** Would it be possible for me to give you some information about allergies and what testing involves, and you could come back in a few weeks to discuss it when you have had a chance to think about it?

Written information
Organising follow-up
Dealing with an inappropriate request and using time as a way to do this

**R:** Yes, that's a good idea. I think I'm in a bit of shock about what happened to Charlie last week.

**D:** Maybe then we can have a longer chat about it and decide how to proceed.

**D:** OK. I'll book to come back and see you in a couple of weeks. Thanks Dr Patel. Have a good weekend.

# Relative scenario 13

| Transcript | Skills demonstrated |
| --- | --- |
| **D:** Good morning Mrs Owens. My name's Dr Jones. Come through. | Used relative's name |
| **R:** Hi there. | |
| **D:** How may I help you today? | Open question |
| **R:** I wanted to talk to you about my husband, Jim Burns. You may want to bring up his notes. | |
| **D:** Can I ask what you wanted to talk about? | |

R: Yes, I just want to check if he's been treated for *Chlamydia.*

D: Before I go any further, I just want to explain that I cannot discuss anything in your husband's records as we have to respect his rights to confidentiality. I know this must be difficult but we can never disclose medical information without having the patient's consent.

**Confidentiality**

R: I understand that but the thing is, I had *Chlamydia* and haven't had sex with anyone apart from my husband for the last 9 years, since we got married. I am worried he may have or at least have given it to me so I really need to know.

D: Have you discussed it with your husband yet?

R: Yes. He denied having it. He said he went and had a test which was negative and tried to brush it off

D: Gosh, it sounds like quite a complicated situation to be in. Would you mind if we could go back to your health at the moment as you said you have been diagnosed with *Chlamydia*. When was this?

R: I went to a walk-in clinic a few weeks ago as I started having pain here and some weird discharge I've never had before. I couldn't believe it as I was sent a note saying I needed this antibiotic and that I needed to contact anyone I have had sex with in the last 6 months to tell them to be treated too.

D: That must have been a huge shock for you. How are you feeling now?

**Empathy**

R: I still have a bit of pain but the discharge has improved. I just feel so dirty.

D: You shouldn't. These sorts of infections are extremely common. Were you tested for anything else?

**Reassurance**

R: Yes, all that was OK. I got tested for everything like HIV and stuff.

D: Have you thought about how you could have got this infection?

**Exploring ideas**

R: I'm sure my husband is having an affair. He must be. I've tried to look at his phone and computer but he doesn't tell me his passwords. It's so frustrating. He's just been ignoring it if I bring up the *Chlamydia*. I am just so angry right now.

D: That sounds extremely difficult and distressing.

R: He tried to have sex with me the other day and I just felt sick. I don't even trust the fact that he's even been tested. Could you just see really quickly and say yes or no to whether he's been tested?

**Empathy**

D: As I said before, I know this is very difficult for you but I really could not do that, as it would be illegal and wrong. I'm really sorry and I know you must be frustrated.

**Being honest and open**

R: OK. I'll try and find out some other way.

D: If your husband is willing to give permission for you to look at his notes that would be different, but that's really the only way I could help you with that. Do you think he would be willing to come in with you to have a discussion, as it seems as if there are quite few issues and we may be able to try and help you work out how to solve this?

**Problem solving**

R: I doubt he would. And he would definitely not allow me to see his notes.

D: Do you think you would want to try something like relationship counselling by someone independent?

**Conceptual thinking**

R: I don't know. There's no way I'm going near Jim now. At least that way he can't give me any infections again.

D: I can understand why you are upset but this is going to destroy your relationship unless you can talk openly to your husband. Most patients who get an infection like yours have acquired it recently but sometimes patients can harbour an infection without any symptoms for years. It's is not something I have a great deal of experience with but I would advise you to speak to someone at the GUM clinic.

**Giving advice for further information and more expert advice**

R: I was thinking of doing that.

D: You could also try again to be open with Jim, explain how you are feeling and how it is affecting you – you certainly can't carry on like this.

R: I know, it is just so hard.

D: I'm really very sorry I cannot do more to help you but I want you to know that I am here to talk at any point if you need to.

R: Thank you.

D: Should we book an appointment in a week or two to discuss how things are going?

Organising follow-up

R: OK, that would be good.

## Relative scenario 14

| Transcript | Skills demonstrated |
| --- | --- |
| D: Hi, good morning Mr. Ward, I am Dr White. How can I help? | Used relative's name |
| R: I'm just quite upset actually. My wife and I are both quite upset. I was tidying my daughter's room and I found the pill. She's only 15! We just don't know what to do. I can't believe she's having sex, I can't believe she's been prescribed the pill. I can't believe the doctors here have given her the pill without asking her parents. It's totally ridiculous! I'm just in shock, she's only 15! | |
| D: I can appreciate that you are very, very upset about this. But I have to explain that I can't specifically discuss your daughter's medical records with you without her consent. | Dealing with anger Confidentiality |
| R: Well, you must be able to, she is only 15, she is still a minor and I have parental responsibility. | |
| D: I can completely understand that you are upset and you feel that you need an explanation. As I said, I can't go into her records and discuss them with you. Would you like me to explain why this is? It may help you to understand the situation a bit better. | Staying calm<br><br>Offering explanation |
| R: I suppose so, OK. | |

**D:** I recognise that she is 15 and that she is a minor, but to maintain that trust with our patients we need to preserve that level of confidentiality, regardless of their age. This is exactly in the same way that I would never discuss your records with anyone else without your consent. As doctors we do have guidelines on dealing with patients who are under 16. I can't say that we have or haven't seen your daughter, but I can explain the process that we go through as doctors if a girl requested contraception. Would that be helpful?

Discussing confidentiality

**R:** Yes – please go ahead.

**D:** If a 15-year-old girl came to ask for the pill, we are trained to assess their level of maturity. We talk at great length about risks and benefits; we also try and encourage them to talk to their parents. However if we do feel that they are mature enough to take the pill, and that they will continue to be sexually active with or without the pill and would therefore put themselves at risk of becoming pregnant, we do prescribe it to them. In other words, we act in their best interests. Does that make sense?

Discussion of Fraser competence

**R:** A bit, so basically what you are saying is that you can't discuss my daughter's case, but if she came in you would try and get her to talk to us and if she doesn't you still give her the pill anyway?

**D:** That is the process we follow for when we see a girl who is under 16 years of age. I know this doesn't help you in how you are feeling. Now that I have explained the process that doctors go through in these situations, would we be able to talk a little bit about how you plan to deal with this from now on?

Signposting

**R:** I think you should stop that prescription, I think she's too young to be having sex.

**D:** Right, as I've said I can't tell you if it has been prescribed or not. I haven't even looked at her notes but I think it may be wise if you and your wife sit down with your daughter, approach her in the first instance and try and discuss it with her and let her know your concerns.

Remaining calm with an angry relative and an unreasonable request

**R:** I think we are going to have to, to be honest.

**D:** I can see that you are quite angry about all of this.

Openly acknowledging relative anger

R: I'm in shock really, she's only a little girl – she shouldn't be having sex. I know she's got a boyfriend, but still.

D: I can completely understand why you are feeling upset and shocked, but it often does help if parents discuss this with their daughter, in a safe environment where she doesn't feel threatened. If you approach it that way she may discuss things openly with you and your wife.

Empathy

R: Yes, I think that is what we will have to do.

D: Again, I'm sorry that I cannot give you more information or assurance that I can do certain things to stop this happening. But we are here to help you, and if you want to come in as a family I am more than happy to discuss it all with you.

R: Thank you, I'm sorry to have wasted your time.

D: No, not at all. You haven't wasted my time.

## Relative scenario 15

| Transcript | Skills demonstrated |
|---|---|
| D: Hi Mr Brett, come in. I'm Dr Hunt. It's good to meet you. | Used relative's name |
| R: Hi Dr Hunt. | |
| D: What can I do for you? | Open question |
| R: I just wanted to talk to you about my wife, Sara. | |
| D: Of course. | |
| R: As you may know, or you might not – I'm not sure really. Anyway, she has cancer … | |
| D: I'm really sorry to hear that. | Empathy |
| R: I know. It's really devastating. | |
| D: I'm sure. [*Pause.*] Can you tell me more about what's going on? | Open question |

R: She's got breast cancer. Or it was just breast cancer and we thought it was all over. She had surgery and chemo and radiotherapy – everything. But it's back and spread everywhere. I don't understand what happened.

D: I'm so sorry to hear that. That sounds terrible for all of you.

Empathy

R: She's so young. And my kids... [*Emotional.*]

D: [*Silence.*] Would you like a glass of water?

Use of silence

R: No. I'm OK.

D: What have the hospital doctors told you about the plan from here?

Exploring understanding

R: They said she is going to have some radiotherapy to her bones in her spine but there's nothing we can do. I have asked them a million times. I thought they could chop it all out but it's in the liver and everywhere now. She's been through so much. It's so unfair. She's just too young to die. All they have really done is put us in touch with the Macmillan team. They are all so good but it makes things seem so negative.

D: And how's Sara coping with it all?

R: She's being amazing. She's had her moments but now she's getting things sorted out and being so matter-of-fact about it all. She's amazing. She's going to think of a way to tell the girls this week. I'm the one who's being ridiculous.

D: What do you mean?

R: I just can't cope with it. I'm a grown man and I don't want them all to think I'm falling apart but I just can't take it. I feel sick to my stomach. I'm not the one who's dying but I feel like I'm falling apart when I need to be strong.

D: You too are going through an absolutely terrible time and it's quite OK to be feeling like this. I don't think anyone in your situation would be feeling any different. How is your health?

Empathy

R: OK. I'm fit and well but I'm not sleeping. I can barely eat, especially as Sara doesn't eat much now. I just watch her in the night and think about the fact that she's only got a few months left. I don't know what I'm going to do without her. Oh dear, that sounds so selfish.

D: You shouldn't think that you should be stronger, or that showing this emotion is a weakness. This is an incredibly difficult time for you, and everybody in your position needs support and help.

Empathy

R: My children need me to be strong, as does Sara, and I am just going to have to get a grip.

D: How old are your children?

R: 7 and 8. They don't know.

D: Have you thought about how you are going to explain things to them?

Picking up on cue

R: No, Sara and I have briefly discussed it but it never seems the right time.

D: It is so hard, and I don't have a great deal of experience with this but I know that the Macmillan team have lots of counsellors that can help, and there is also lot of written information available which explains how such things can be explained to children.

R: Well yes, Jen our Macmillan nurse is really good and she's been trying to get us all to see their counsellor but I don't feel ready for it yet.

D: I see. You mentioned you are struggling to sleep at the moment. Is this something you feel you may want help with, in terms of medication?

Reflecting back on something previously disclosed

R: No. I'm OK for now but thanks.

D: Do you have a good support network who knows about the situation?

R: Yes, our closest friends all know and they are going to help me with the kids, especially their godparents. My family live in New Zealand but Sara's parents and sister are around. They know what's going on and are in a bit of a state right now as well. Sara's mum keeps coming over and trying to force her to eat as she thinks that's the most important thing. It's a bit annoying for Sara, as the poor thing just doesn't want to be harassed. We know she means well though.

D: It sounds as though you have a lot of people around you who care. I think you've done a really good thing coming here today. We are also here to help you with any problems that come along.

R: Thank you.

D: Are you working at the moment?

R: Yes, I'm an architect. Everyone's has been incredible though. They know and have told me I can take time off whenever I need to. They're great. I try to get on with things as I don't want to stay home and pity myself all the time as it's not me that's dying.

Exploring impact of illness – think home, relationships, finances, work

D: I understand you wanting to keep busy but it's OK to feel like that – you are all going through a time of huge strain and pressure. If you do need a few days off I would not hesitate to take it.

R: I know. I will if I think I need to or when Sara needs me, then of course.

D: You are going through a terrible time at the moment and I know you feel that you need to stay strong for Sara and your children but you mustn't feel that needing help and support yourself is a weakness. You are going to need a great deal of support and I can't see that trying to soldier on and do everything by yourself is a very good option. You sound as though you are being incredibly supportive and that your family is lucky to have you, but please think about taking some time out each day to look after yourself.

Empathy, reassurance and encouragement

R: I know you are right doctor, and I do feel better for just having spoken to you. Do you think we should see the counsellor?

**D:** Well, yes. Patients in the past have said that it is very useful and I would have thought it would be worth a try.

**R:** OK, I'll talk to Sara about it.

**D:** Do you want to come back, maybe even with Sara for another chat sometime and maybe to discuss getting you some extra support for the kids?

Organising follow-up

**R:** Yes, that would be great. I'll have to check the diary as we've got so many appointments with the hospital in the next week, but I'll book in again soon. Thanks.

**D:** Is there anything else you wanted to talk about today?

**R:** No, I'm fine. Thanks Dr Hunt.

**D:** I wish you all the best and please do book in whenever you want. If you find it difficult to fit in coming here you can also call me if you want to discuss anything or leave a message and I'll call you back.

Being understanding and flexible about access to contacting you

**R:** I will. Thank you.

# Healthcare professional scenario 1

| Transcript | Skills demonstrated |
|---|---|
| **D:** Good morning Sue. Come through. | Used colleague's name |
| **H:** Thank you very much for agreeing to talk to me today. | |
| **D:** That's fine. How can I help? | Open question |
| **H:** I just wanted to talk to you about a few problems I've been having lately and I really wanted to get some advice from somebody who is neutral to the situation, I hope you don't mind me speaking to you. | |
| **D:** No, not at all, I hope I can help. | Encouraging contribution |
| **H:** Well, the ward sister Jane has been doing things lately that have been upsetting me. | |
| **D:** I'm sorry to hear that. What has been happening? | Open question |
| **H:** Loads of stuff really. I mean the worst thing is she's been making me do jobs that no one else wants to do. For example, I do know I'm supposed to be doing things like cleaning patients who vomit or soil themselves, but if there are loads of us around to do things, it's always me that she'll ask. She's not giving me the chance to do other things I find more useful, like putting in lines or doing the medications. Now I just feel like I'm being held back here. I've worked hard and I am a band 4 nurse. I just don't feel that I make enough progress. | |
| **D:** It sounds as though you've had a difficult time lately and I'm sorry to see that you're so upset. Have you felt that she's always been like this with you? | Empathy |
| **H:** No. What I'm most sad about it is the fact we used to get on very well. We had a real laugh together and she was always helping me out. I always looked up to her as I think she's an excellent nurse herself. I was learning lots from her and it was generally great in the department. I really enjoyed working in A&E. | |
| **D:** Do you have any thoughts as to why your relationship may have changed? | Exploring ideas |

**H:** Something happened a few months ago and I think that is probably why she changed the way she is with me.

**D:** Do you want to tell me what happened?

Open question

**H:** Well, I saw her give the wrong medication to a patient so I approached her about it at the time. She seemed fine and we had a chat about it but I then filled out an incident form. We had to have a talk about it within the department and speak to the line manager and things, but everything looked like it was all sorted out in the end. I thought she agreed that I should do that as this is what I've always been taught – that's what we're supposed to do! I've seen her do that herself when doctors have made mistakes.

**D:** Do you mind me asking what happened and if anyone came to serious harm?

Ensuring safety

**H:** No, that's fine. She gave a patient paracetamol who was in the wrong bed. It was a string of things that happened and it was not entirely her fault because the drug chart was by that wrong patient's bed. So I really didn't feel that I acted in a way that was blaming her at all and I don't think I was persecutory in anyway. But obviously she felt differently. I think it's because she has never made a mistake before and is a bit of a perfectionist. I think she was quite affected by it.

**D:** It sounds like it's been a difficult time for you. You said that you feel she is giving you the worst jobs and unfairly penalising you. Have you noticed anything else happening?

Empathy, reflecting back and exploring further

**H:** Well, it's got to a point where we're not even really speaking. We used to go after work for drinks with the other guys. We were all quite close. Now she just doesn't invite me anywhere and talks about their nights out in front of me. She won't even say hello to me in the morning. It really has got to a point where I feel like I can't talk to her. Yesterday, for example, she screamed at me in front of everyone for being 10 minutes late. I'm always early to work but what can I do if the tube is delayed by 40 minutes?

**D:** No, that is not appropriate. You said before you think she's an excellent nurse. Have you any concerns about her clinical work?

**H:** No, I don't think so. I think that this may have been a one-off. I've never seen her make any other mistakes. She is normally very diligent but I think that she finds it difficult to accept blame or fault.

**D:** I understand that you feel rather singled out – have you ever noticed her behaving like this to anyone else?

**H:** I suppose she has been rude about some of the doctors, but then again we all get annoyed at people at work. I don't think she's singled anyone out in the way she's doing to me right now.

**D:** I'm really glad that you have come to talk to me about the situation because I can see that you're having a very difficult time at the moment. Do you feel that the other nurses are treating you in this way as well?

**H:** Yes, in a way. I feel that they want to impress Jane because she's so senior and has been in the department for so long. It's kind of like they know that she doesn't want them to involve me so they feel they have to behave in the same way. It just got out of control in this place.

**D:** Do you think it is affecting your performance in any way at work?

Impact on work, home, relationships

**H:** Well, as I said before I feel like I'm not getting a chance to progress and I don't get a chance to keep my skills up. But apart from that I try to get on with things and work hard.

**D:** And is this affecting you when you are outside of work?

**H:** It does – everyday. I must say I've been coming home and my boyfriend is just so fed up at the moment because as I've been talking about things every night. I've even cried a few nights and it sounds silly but it really has been getting me down. I don't how much more you can take. I don't even want to do anything after work or go out anymore.

**D:** It sounds like this is affecting you quite badly. Have you spoken to anyone apart from your boyfriend about this?

**H:** Initially I was speaking to my friends but at the moment I can't be bothered to meet anyone or go out and do anything so I don't really see them very much.

**D:** It really does sound like this is affecting you. Some of the things you are describing sound as though you may be suffering from depression. Have you thought about that?

**H:** Yeah definitely. I mean, I've lost weight and I am not eating much. I've been reading about depression and I think I do have it. I bet my boyfriend thinks I do too as I'm just such an awful person to be around lately.

**D:** Have you thought about speaking to your GP about this?

**H:** It's so difficult to get an appointment these days and get time off but I suppose I could go after a night shift next week.

**D:** There are also counsellors available within the occupational health department. It might be worth seeing if you can speak to somebody there.

**H:** That could be a good idea.

**D:** You mentioned before that your boyfriend is concerned about you and you feel you're not good to be around. Is everything OK at home?

**H:** Oh yes, that's been fine. He's really great and we've been together for years and years and he is really trying to help me. There is only so much you can do though. He just keeps telling me to leave work and do something else. I suppose he would probably be happy if I did a different job and didn't always have to do long shifts and weekends.

**D:** I just want to let you know that there are people like myself available to talk if things do get worse. But I would really encourage you to see your own GP.

**H:** Thank you.

**D:** Thinking back to the problems at work that have probably caused all of this, did you have any ideas about how these issues could be resolved?

**H:** The only thing I thought about is leaving my job. I've looked at my contract – I've got a 2-month notice period so I was thinking of just moving to a new department or applying to a different hospital.

**D:** Is this something you feel that you will have to do?

**H:** Well, it's not what I want ideally because it's so convenient for me to get here. But if things carry on like this it's probably the best thing. It just feels like a bit of déjà vu really.

**D:** What do you mean by that?

Picking up on cue

**H:** I had the same problem at school when I was 13. There were some really horrible girls in my class who bullied me. I remember this went on for a couple of years and it really upset me and affected my family as well. I ended up leaving then and I was so much happier in my new school, so I guess this is why I feel like there is no other option than to leave.

**D:** Is there anything you were hoping that I could do for you specifically?

Exploring expectations

**H:** Well, I don't know really. I just wanted to talk to somebody about it who isn't directly involved in the situation.

**D:** I'm really pleased that you have spoken to me about everything. I can totally understand why you feel that you want to leave but, on the other hand, it seems a shame if you were previously very happy here. Have you thought about ways to try and make things better by talking to Jane and the other nursing staff?

Empathy and sensitivity

**H:** I don't really see how I'm going to do that.

**D:** It sounds like this is a form of bullying and that you are being treated most unfairly. First of all, it would probably be best to have a meeting with Jane to try to get everything out in the open. If she realised how she was making you feel and how upset you were, she may want to resolve the matter.

**H:** That's probably a good idea but I'm sure she is aware of how upset I am. I can only imagine things getting worse.

**D:** It is important to ensure that people realise bullying is not acceptable in any environment so, although it may seem that the easy thing to do would be to ignore things, it is better in the long run to try and change things. This is not only for you but also for others in the future as well. If they did realise the seriousness of the situation and potential consequences it may change their behaviour. Is there anyone more senior than Jane you feel you could talk to in the department if meeting Jane didn't work?

> Problem solving and explanation about not tolerating bullying at work

**H:** Yes, there is our line manager and another senior sister. She is not really involved on the wards as she does a lot of admin work but I suppose I could talk to her. I don't want to be seen as a troublemaker because if I do apply for a new job I will need a decent reference.

**D:** The best-case scenario would be to try and resolve things amongst yourselves, especially with Jane in first instance. But if you feel you can't, and things are getting worse it is always worth taking things further then. How do you feel about that?

**H:** I think you are right. I won't look forward to it but I will try to arrange a meeting with Jane.

**D:** Good. Would it be possible to meet again at some point to see how things are going? Maybe in a few days time?

> Organising follow-up

**H:** Of course, I'd like that.

**D:** OK, and I would also once again encourage you to see your GP.

**H:** Yes, I think you're right. I'll definitely go and see my GP. I do feel a bit better already just to have got this off my chest.

**D:** Good, I'll be around the department so please do feel free to come and have a chat with me and I'll keep my eyes out to see if I can pick up on anything as well. It may be worth jotting down things in a diary if anything happens from now on, in case you don't manage to resolve things and do need to take this further.

**H:** I think you're right. Thanks for your help.

## Healthcare professional scenario 2

| Transcript | Skills demonstrated |
|---|---|
| **D:** Hi Lizzie. Come on in. | Used colleague's name |
| **D:** You look upset. | Recognising emotion |
| **H:** I just feel so awful, it's just been a really bad day. You're going to think I'm really silly! I'm so sorry to cry. | |
| **D:** That's OK. Take your time. | Use of silence |
| **H:** I'm just so upset today about poor Mr Franks. He died this morning and I know you're going to think I'm being really silly but it's just the way he died – it was so awful. | |
| **D:** Could you tell me a little bit more about what happened? | Open question |
| **H:** I just don't know if there's anything that could have been done to him to make him feel better. I mean, I was trying to do his physiotherapy every day and he was just such a lovely man and was so grateful for everything that we did for him. It just feels like he was so uncomfortable all the time and always so breathless. You must think this is so silly. I'm so embarrassed. | |
| **D:** No, not at all. You shouldn't be embarrassed and I can understand why you'd feel this way. How long have you been feeling like this for? | Empathy |
| **H:** Well, I've been upset since I started looking after him because I really wanted him to be OK. Don't get me wrong, I knew he was ill and I knew he was never going to be well but he was just so young. He was only 55. It's just so horrible. | |
| **D:** [*Pause*] I do agree it is always really difficult when people die and you're not alone in getting upset about it. Some patients do tend to affect you more than others. Are you generally finding it difficult in this job? | Use of silence |
| **H:** I don't know. I have been doing my oncology placement for a month now and it isn't the easiest job. I do actually really enjoy it, but this sort of thing gets me down quite a lot. I have been okay with other people so I just don't know why Mr Franks has affected me like this. | |

D: Have you spoken to anyone else about how you're feeling, apart from me?

H: No, I don't want them to feel like I'm being silly and overdramatic.

D: Do you think that there's any particular reason why Mr Franks has affected you so much?

**Exploring ideas**

H: I don't know. I suppose it's just his age. It's probably brought back some horrible memories as well.

D: Would you mind me asking what it's reminded you of?

**Picking up on cue**

H: My mum died about 5 years ago. She was quite unwell. She had pancreatic cancer. And I was told that the doctors would do everything to make her feel comfortable but she never was. She had a horrible death too – she was vomiting until the end and we never really got on top of her pain. It was just awful.

D: I'm sorry to hear that. It sounds like it's been really tough on you. Did you say that was 5 years ago?

**Empathy**
**Clarifying facts**

H: Yes.

D: Well, I can see why this job has been difficult for you considering what you've experienced in the past. How are you feeling now about your mum's death?

H: I feel OK as I've had some time to deal it but things like this do remind me of her.

D: And how are the rest of your family?

H: They're OK. I've only got my dad and he lives nearby. It's been a little bit difficult because he was quite dependent on my mum and this all came as such a shock to all of us really. She died within about 5 months of being diagnosed. He's trying to cope but he's on his own now and I worry about him. He's barely spoken about mum.

D: That sounds very difficult. Have you talked to anyone at home about your job?

**Exploring support network**

H: My husband's been brilliant since she died and since I started this job. We have spoken about a few things. I don't really like to bring work home with me.

D: I understand that. Do you feel that you may need to get extra support because of what's happened and because of the nature of the job you are doing at the moment?

H: No, I think I'll be OK. Maybe the more stuff like this I see the easier it will get.

D: That's definitely possible. But what if it does not get easier?

H: I suppose I could speak to someone. I feel a lot better just now having spoken about everything.

D: This is a difficult job and today has probably been more difficult because of all the memories that it's brought back. It is quite natural to feel like this and I don't want you to be embarrassed about talking to me. I'm sure a lot of your colleagues would be more than understanding and may even have been feeling the same as you before. I know I have felt very emotional about some of my patients in the past.

Reassurance and bringing in personal experience

H: Thank you.

D: Do you think you're going to be OK to carry on working today? It may be worth speaking to your supervisor to see if you can go home.

Ensuring safe to work

H: Oh no! I think I'll be OK. I think I just needed to get it out of my system really.

D: Thank you for coming to speak to me about it today. Is there anything you think I can do for you to help you?

H: No, thank you for listening though. I just wanted to tell someone how I was feeling.

D: If you don't feel that you want to talk to your colleagues I'm obviously around if you want to grab me from time to time. It may also be worth speaking to someone about your mum and may be getting some counselling? What are your thoughts about that?

H: I could do that but I think I'll see how I go.

D: Of course, is there anything else you wanted to talk about?

**H:** No, I'm fine. I think I'll have a quick cup of tea and then get back to work. Thank you for being so kind and for talking to me today.

**D:** That's no problem. If you feel that you want to speak to me again today you know my bleep number. I'll be around this afternoon.

Organising follow-up

# Healthcare professional scenario 3

| Transcript | Skills demonstrated |
| --- | --- |
| **D:** Hi Karen, come on in. | Used colleague's name |
| **H:** Thank you Dr Hall. | |
| **D:** How can I help? | Open question |
| **H:** Thanks for taking the time to talk to me today. I just wanted to have a word with you about Dr Dias. | |
| **D:** Of course, what did you want to discuss? | |
| **H:** I just had a few concerns about him, I'm not sure if you've noticed? He's just been very short-tempered with us and really hasn't been doing very well at work recently. | Open question |
| **D:** Well, thanks for coming and speaking to me, I know it can take a lot to do that and I'm sorry to hear he has been short-tempered with you. What sort of things has been going on? | Empathy<br>Encouragement |
| **H:** I'm sure other staff must have noticed. He has been arriving late at least three times a week, he has been forgetting to do the prescriptions and he has started to run really late with his surgeries. Patients keep coming to the desk to complain about being kept waiting and I've overheard a few patients saying that he was really rude with them. He also keeps coming in looking very scruffy. I mean, yesterday it looked as though he had been wearing the same shirt all week! | |
| **D:** Dr Dias has been with us for a few months, so how long have you noticed this going on for? | |
| **H:** He was fine when he first started. I think it's been going on over the past 3 or 4 weeks, and it's just been getting worse. | Clarifying history of the problem |

**D:** And have you noticed anything else?

**H:** Not really – he just seems so annoyed all of the time.

**D:** OK, there certainly seems to be something going on. Have you seen any occasions where patients have been put at risk by his behaviour?

Checking patient safety

**H:** I don't think so, but loads have been inconvenienced – having to return again to pick up scripts and things like that.

**D:** Well, thank you for telling me about this. It does seem strange that his performance and behaviour would change so dramatically. I wonder whether there is anything going on outside work that is affecting him or maybe he is finding the role too stressful.

Verbalising thoughts

**H:** Yes, that is what I was wondering.

**D:** Did you have any ideas about the best way forward?

Exploring ideas

**H:** I just don't want to cause trouble. I know what it's like, you start talking about people and things get out of hand. I don't know really, I'd have normally spoken to his trainer but he is away for a few weeks so you were my next port of call. Maybe you could have a word with him?

**D:** I agree that would be the best idea. I think it's got to a point where something does need to be done.

**H:** Yes, that would be great.

**D:** I'll try to speak to him tomorrow but I'll also feed back to his trainer when he returns from holiday. I'm very keen to ensure that his performance improves. Will you let me know if you have any more concerns in the future?

Organising follow-up

**H:** That would be great. Thanks again for listening.

**D:** No problem.

# Healthcare professional scenario 4

| Transcript | Skills demonstrated |
|---|---|
| **D:** Good morning Kate, come in. | Used colleague's name |
| **H:** Thank you Dr Constable. | |
| **D:** I had a message saying you wanted to talk to me? | |
| **H:** Yes, thank you. I really wanted to chat to you about something that happened last week at work. | |
| **D:** Of course. | |
| **H:** I'm a bit worried to be honest and I don't want it to get around that I've reported this – you will keep it discreet won't you? | |
| **D:** Yes. I will certainly try and handle anything you tell me discreetly and sensitively. Would you be able to tell me a little bit about what happened? | Open question |
| **H:** Yes. It's just about Dr Iredale. I was in the middle of a shift in A&E and he was seeing an elderly Indian lady who had quite a lot of medical issues and was struggling to explain herself. He came and sat down and loudly said in front of everybody: 'I wish these people would just go back to their own country. How come they can't even learn English? They shouldn't be allowed to live here if they can't speak the language.' | |
| **D:** Oh dear, that's completely unacceptable. Thank you for telling me this. What happened after that? | Quickly reassuring your colleague that you have recognised the seriousness of the problem |
| **H:** Well, I walked away and didn't really say anything. I was so shocked. I haven't said or done anything about it since then. | |
| **D:** Was anyone else there at the time that heard these comments? | |
| **H:** I think one of the nurses, Clare, was there and she was talking to another doctor. I don't know that doctor's name though, but I think she was from the medical team. | |
| **D:** And have you ever heard any other comments like this before? | |

H: No, I haven't heard anything else like this before. Once was enough. I left straightaway as I couldn't really sit and listen to it anymore.

D: You are right. This is very concerning. Have you had any thoughts about what you want to do?

Exploring ideas

H: I would love to complain, which is the reason I've come to you today. It's really been bothering me. I have spoken to my family about this and they said I can't just let it go but I don't want to get a bad reputation in this department as I'm just a healthcare assistant and am worried that people won't believe me.

D: I would hate to think that no one would believe you or take you seriously. Is that the main thing that you worried about?

Picking up on cue

H: Well no, that's not all. Something happened a few months ago where a nurse reported another nurse who gave the wrong fluids to a patient. She was treated so badly afterwards that she ended up leaving because nobody could trust her after that. I know what people think about whistleblowing. I really need this job as I want to start nursing at some point and I just can't afford to lose it really.

D: I understand your concerns but that should never happen. There are policies and procedures in place to ensure that people who raise concerns aren't penalised in any way. Would you consider telling anyone else about this?

Providing reassurances based on a specific concerns

H: I'd hate to, I really would. Could you deal with things for me?

D: From what you've said it really does sound like what happened was unacceptable. Racism is something that should never be tolerated. It's difficult reporting this sort of thing second hand. I suppose I could ask to see Dr Iredale and explain that he was overheard making these comments but it would be difficult to take it much further.

Verbalising thoughts on how to deal with this issue

H: I'd really appreciate that. I think if I knew that somebody was doing something about it I'd feel a lot better. I just feel that the same thing coming from a healthcare assistant in this department could not carry very much weight.

D: I don't want you to feel that you're not valued here as every member of this team is important. Your opinion and your feelings are just as important as anybody else's. I hope I can reassure you of that. Are you worried about anything else Dr Iredale has done or said?

*Picking up on cue*

*Encouraging colleague*

H: No, not really. I would like it if you could speak to him though, at least then he would know that he had been heard and that you thought it was wrong.

D: Yes, it would be a start. Would you mind if I also spoke to my consultant to get advice. I wouldn't have to mention your name.

H: That would be OK, I think.

D: I'm really glad you bought this to my attention and I know that you are very worried about how it will affect your reputation. I am sorry you feel that you can't be open because that really shouldn't be how anyone should feel. I think it's important that you're kept up-to-date with what's going on. Do you want to arrange to meet me in a couple of weeks when I've had a chance to speak to Dr Iredale and my consultant?

*Organising follow-up*

H: That's fine.

D: OK. Well, thank you very much for speaking to me. This is a really important issue and you were absolutely correct to have raised it.

## Healthcare professional scenario 5

| Transcript | Skills demonstrated |
| --- | --- |
| D: Hello Bill, come in. | Used colleague's name |

H: Thanks for agreeing to talk to me.

D: That's no problem at all. Sorry we couldn't speak yesterday.

**H:** That's OK. I really just wanted a chat with you about a couple of things. Um, well, you may know I've been in this department for a while, in fact a good 15 years so I consider myself to be very experienced. But I've got a few concerns about our new consultant, Mr Blackbridge.

**D:** What sort of concerns do you have?

> Open question

**H:** I don't know if you've noticed anything yourself but the infection rate in this department has gone up massively since Mr Blackbridge started. I've noticed the postop wound infection rates are very high.

**D:** OK, this is very important. Do you have any particular thoughts as to what he might be doing to cause this?

> Exploring ideas

**H:** Nothing's changed from our perspective. The nursing staff are the same and we have been cleaning wounds and people are getting their prophylactic antibiotics. So my gut feeling is that something must be happening during the operations.

**D:** Apart from the infection rates is there anything else that you worried about with Mr Blackbridge?

> Gathering all of the information before coming up with a plan

**H:** Sort of – yes. I am concerned about the way he behaves and the fact that he is quite rude to some of my junior nurses, and I've seen him being a bit rude to junior doctors. He is fine with me as he's never said anything directly but when I have tried to say to him that I am concerned about some of his patients he sort of breezed over this and asked me to talk to his registrar. I do feel that I'm kind of being ignored.

**D:** Can you think of specific examples about what he's been doing?

**H:** Well, I mean, I said to him that a patient has got a wound infection this afternoon and I was so surprised that he said 'why are you telling me? Call my house officer' and didn't even really care or want to see the patient after their operation.

**D:** That sounds quite frustrating for you.

> Empathy

**H:** There was also another incident. I was worried about one of his patients who was breathless after a hip replacement. I mentioned this to him and he just said 'speak to the SHO' and then walked off. I feel like he just leaves everything to his juniors to sort out. Most patients he's operated on don't ever meet him before of after. He never even consents the patients.

**D:** Do you think the other consultants do things very differently?

**H:** Yes. As I said I have been here for 15 years and I have always worked with very good consultants and have had no concerns about any of them.

**D:** From what you're saying it sounds quite serious and we should really investigate this matter. Have you talked to anyone else about this?

Reassuring colleague that you are taking this seriously

**H:** No. I don't really want to be the bad guy but at the same time I know I've got a duty to report this. Or at least try and make things better. I am very protective about this whole department and it just isn't running the way it should do with this high infection rate.

**D:** Have you had any ideas about how I could help you in this situation?

Exploring ideas and expectations

**H:** I just want someone to take this matter on, or at least help me do it.

**D:** I'm really pleased that you have felt that you could talk to me about this and it does sound as though things have deteriorated in the department, from what you're saying. It looks like patients are coming to harm so it definitely does need to be investigated.

Patient care at risk

**H:** Good, I feel a bit better having got it off my chest.

**D:** I must say that I am not entirely sure of the best way to proceed. Something definitely needs to be done but I am not convinced that I should approach Mr Blackbridge directly. It may be better coming from another consultant. Would you be happy for me to discuss this with one of the other surgical consultants?

Dealing with difficult situations

Seeking senior help

**H:** Yes, that would be fine.

**D:** Another option would be to talk to the infection control team in the hospital and see whether they have noticed any patterns of infection. We certainly need to do something about this quickly and try to do something in order to minimise further risks to patients.

Verbalising thoughts

**H:** OK, I could do that. I know them well.

**D:** It may also be worth doing an audit to look at complication rates in patients in the department to get some proper evidence about whether rates are different amongst different consultants. It is, of course, important to remember that there are many factors affecting a surgeon's complication rates. I don't know anything about Mr Blackbridge's cases but some patients are more prone to infections than others, irrespective of surgical skill and the like.

Keeping an open mind

**H:** That's a really good idea.

**D:** You also mentioned earlier that Mr Blackbridge is not seeing his postoperative patients and has been rude to staff on occasions. These are very important issues and I will raise them when I speak to my consultant for advice. In the meantime, if there are any further things that happen you could write them up as significant event analyses so they can be looked into further. You could also fill in some incident forms.

Reflecting back

**H:** I have done a few incident forms already but I'll definitely keep a note of things now.

**D:** I know we are pressed for time today and we have discussed quite a lot. Could I just summarise what we've been talking about?

Signposting

**H:** Yes.

**D:** You have raised two important concerns. Firstly, Mr Blackbridge is not seeing his patients postoperatively and possibly has higher infection rates. Secondly, his general attitude in the ward towards staff. We've talked about some possible solutions to this problem and you are happy for me to get some advice from my consultant at this point.

Summarising

H: Yes, that sounds great.

D: Shall we meet again in a few days just to see how things are going and I can let you know when I've spoken to my consultant.

H: Yup, that's fine.

| | Organising follow-up |
|---|---|

## Healthcare professional scenario 6

| Transcript | Skills demonstrated |
|---|---|
| D: Hello Jenny. Do come in. | Used colleague's name |
| H: Oh hi James – thanks for agreeing to speak to me. Sorry if I sounded stressed when I asked you to speak to me earlier. | |
| D: That's OK. How can I help? | Open question |
| H: I just wanted to run something past you that happened last week. I went to use the printer in the doctors' office as we had a problem with the one on the ward. I found one of the consultants, Dr Thomas, kissing his new FY1, Stephanie. It was so awkward and just so embarrassing for us all. | |
| D: I can imagine. What happened after that? | Empathy and open question |
| H: I apologised initially and just left but since then Dr Thomas has come up to me and asked me to be discreet about the situation. I just don't really know what to do now. | |
| D: OK, I can understand why you are stressed about it. Has anything else happened since that day? | |
| H: Well, Stephanie just avoids eye contact with me and I have seen her around the wards quite a lot. She's obviously very upset or embarrassed. Dr Thomas is just behaving as normal and has been really nice. He hasn't mentioned anything again. | |
| D: Is there anything else that you're worried about specifically? | Trying to get all the information early on in the consultation |

**H:** I don't mean to be judgemental, as I know this sort of thing happens all the time but Dr Thomas is married with children so I don't like knowing the fact that he is having an affair, but I know it's none of my business really. I suppose they are both adults and they can do whatever they want to do, but I don't think that it should happen at hospital in the doctors' office.

**D:** I agree. That is a very important point. Were they supposed to be working at the time?

**H:** Oh yes. Stephanie was on-call and she was the medical FY1. It's not really very professional.

**D:** No it is not. Do you think that their relationship may have been affecting their work in any way?

**H:** I can sense Stephanie is feeling a bit uncomfortable around me at the moment and, although Dr Thomas spoke to me before, I have no other complaints about him. I had noticed Dr Thomas and Stephanie joking around a lot and being rather flirty when they was doing those online assessment things together.

**D:** Is Dr Thomas Stephanie's supervisor?

Picking up on cues

**H:** I think so, I can't imagine that's particularly fair.

**D:** I can see why you are a bit worried – that is a bit concerning.

**H:** I honestly don't know what to do. I've been having a few sleepless nights thinking about what to do.

**D:** It's a very difficult situation so I can understand why you're feeling like that. From what you're saying it sounds as though Stephanie and Dr Thomas may also be quite stressed about it. Have you had some ideas yourself about what you could do?

Empathy

Exploring ideas

**H:** I've thought of confronting Dr Thomas and just being honest and saying I think it's inappropriate, but I don't feel like I can. That's why I thought I would run it past someone neutral to get some ideas myself.

**D:** My feeling is that there are several issues here. Firstly, I'm glad it's not affected your working relationship with Dr Thomas but then again it seems things have been difficult for both you and Stephanie on the ward if she is avoiding eye contact and things like that. Maybe it would be good if you both spoke about what happened to make sure she is feeling OK at work and that it is not affecting her.

*Reflecting back earlier conversation*

**H:** Yes, I suppose.

**D:** The other issue that you've raised is quite serious and that's about the fact that Dr Thomas is filling out assessment forms for Stephanie. If they are having a personal relationship this may lead to prejudice and affect his assessment of her. It would probably be more appropriate if someone else were doing them for her.

*Verbalising thoughts*

**H:** That's what I suspected.

**D:** Having relationships in working hours and in the doctors' office seems unprofessional. Would you feel comfortable speaking to Stephanie and Dr Thomas about this matter or would you prefer if someone else had a word with them about it?

*Coming up with potential solutions*

**H:** He's already asked me to be discreet about it so I don't know really. I think it would be good if I spoke to Stephanie. I wouldn't really know how to bring up the assessment things to a senior consultant though.

**D:** I can understand that this could be difficult. I'm not entirely sure about the rules and regulations of this sort of thing and it might be helpful if I spoke to my medical defence union and got some confidential advice about what you've told me today and how best to proceed. I could then speak to you again once I know this. Does that sound reasonable?

*Empathy
Honesty*

*Seeking appropriate help and advice*

**H:** Yes, that would be great because I'm not sure really where I stand with this.

**D:** I'm quite happy to do that this week and in the meantime if you are happy speaking to Stephanie that would be a good starting point. Could we meet next week when we've both have a chance to do these things and then talk again?

*Organising follow-up*

**H:** Yes, that's fine.

**D:** I know this has been a very stressful situation at the moment but is this affecting you in any other way? You mentioned you have had some sleepless nights?

Reflecting back

**H:** I have. Apart from this I'm fine. I have mentioned it all to my fiancé but he just laughed at me and told me to ignore it and let people do what they want.

**D:** Well, I'm pleased you felt you could talk to me and obviously I can assure you that I won't tell anyone what we have spoken of yet until I have further advice, as it's important we remain discreet about the situation to avoid unnecessary embarrassment and gossip.

Professionalism

**H:** Exactly.

**D:** Is there anything else you wanted to mention?

**H:** No. Thank you.

## Healthcare professional scenario 7

| Transcript | Skills demonstrated |
|---|---|
| **D:** Hi Caroline. Do come in. | Used colleague's name |
| **H:** Thank you. | |
| **D:** How can I help? | Open question |
| **H:** I just hoped I could have a word with you really. Sort of as a representative for the rest of your colleagues. | |
| **D:** Of course, what did you want to talk to me about? | Open question |
| **H:** I've been working down here in the lab for quite some time – almost 5 years, and in the last 6 months since the new junior doctors started, things have been more difficult for us. We've been getting a lot of blood samples sent down with completely inadequate labelling of blood bottles. | |
| **D:** I'm sorry to hear that. Can you tell me a bit more about what you have noticed? | Empathy, open question |

H: Well, the samples are coming through with smudged writing so you can't read anything on the bottles. We also get many without a date of birth or hospital number. We just cannot legally process these samples without adequate information. We've also had a few instances where the wrong samples are put with the wrong forms and again there's nothing that we can do apart from discard those samples, so it really has been a bit of a problem now.

D: OK, thank you for raising this issue. Something definitely needs to be done. You mentioned that it seems to have been occurring over the past 6 months. Have you noticed any specific patterns of doctors mislabelling bottles?

Gathering appropriate information

H: It's mainly an issue from the surgical wards. I just come to work expecting the arguments now.

D: What arguments are those?

Picking up on cue

H: Oh, it's not uncommon for doctors to shout at us for not processing the bloods. It's not nice. I mean I know it must be frustrating but people should treat their colleagues with respect.

D: Absolutely – that is right and I am sorry you have been subjected to that.

Empathy

H: I know it is bad when samples can't be processed and patients have to be re-bled but I'd have thought the doctors would have learned.

D: This is very important and I am glad you have brought this to my attention. Patient care is being put at risk, at the very least patients are having to be bled twice and at worst there may be a delay in diagnosis and management.

Appreciating impact upon patients

H: Yes I know. I just really need this to be sorted out

D: I'm sorry that this is been happening and I apologise if I have sent any myself and also on behalf of my colleagues. Is there anything you thought of that I could be able to help you with to resolve this matter?

Exploring ideas and expectations

H: I just want this to be relayed to the junior doctors, especially those on the surgical wards. It would be really helpful if you could educate them in some way as to how to label bottles.

**D:** I think that is a good idea. Maybe I should put some posters up in the doctors' mess and also raise this issue at our next educational meeting.

Making suggestions

**H:** That would be good.

**D:** Could you also keep a note of particular incidents in future in case I need to speak to doctors individually? Perhaps we could do an audit to present at a departmental meeting to show where the problems lie.

**H:** That's quite a good idea. I hadn't really thought of that.

**D:** We have also discussed people being rude to you over the phone. I will certainly talk to my colleagues and reiterate that this is not acceptable but please don't hesitate to contact me should there be any further instances.

Reflecting back

**H:** Thank you so much. You've been really helpful.

**D:** OK, so would you mind if I summarised what we have talked about.

Signposting

**H:** Not at all.

**D:** There has been an emerging pattern of mislabelled blood bottles coming from the surgical wards especially. This leads to the samples being rejected, patients being re-bled and on some occasions, doctors being very rude down the phone. First of all we have agreed that I will speak to my colleagues, and everyone is aware of the labelling requirements and that it is unacceptable to be rude to colleagues. We have also agreed to keep a record of any future incidents so that we could do an audit if the need arose.

Summarising

**H:** That is great – thank you.

# Healthcare professional scenario 8

| Transcript | Skills demonstrated |
|---|---|
| **D:** Hello Mrs Walsh, come in. | Used colleague's name |
| **D:** How are you? | |
| **H:** Not bad. I was just hoping to have a quick word with you about one of the FY1s, Dr Peters. | |
| **D:** Of course. | |
| **H:** Right, where can I start? I'm just basically a little worried about him. | |
| **D:** OK, can you tell me what you're worried about? | Open question |
| **H:** Well, he's been here for a few months now and I understand that he's still very new but I have had a couple of experiences with him that have caused me a little bit of concern. I'm not sure what everybody else thinks but I've been on call with him on a few weekends and I just think that he is not coping at work. | |
| **D:** OK, what have you noticed? | Open question |
| **H:** I appreciate the fact that he asks for help and I like it when junior doctors do that. But he seems to be asking for advice about the same sort of thing all the time. He is also leaving my patients so bruised after trying multiple cannulas on those with good veins. I'm just not sure if he's quite ready to be working on his own. He just seems to be very stressed. | |
| **D:** Have you felt concerned about any of the other FY1s? | |
| **H:** Well no, and that's the thing. I have been here for so long and seen so many FY1s come and go and no one I have come across has struggled like this. | |
| **D:** That sounds worrying and I can see you are very concerned about it. Could you be more specific about things he is not learning and also if anything has happened to a patient as a result of his care? | Empathy<br>Gathering important information |

**H:** He just keeps asking the nursing staff how much fluid to give a patient and which one. More worryingly, there was a postop patient who had a low urine output and he didn't really seem to know the basic first steps to take. He was just asking us what he should do.

**D:** What happened then?

**H:** I suggested he ought to take blood tests to make sure the patient wasn't anaemic. I eventually ended up bleeping the on-call SHO who came down and sorted things out. I was really quite worried for this patient because Dr Peters seemed to panic and not actually do anything.

**D:** That sounds serious. Have you had any other experiences with him where patients may have been at risk?

Ensuring patient safety

**H:** It's only really when you see him on call that this sort of thing happens. Usually in the week there are lots of other doctors who are there to help out, which is great, but I do see him struggling in the day with general decision-making. Even for little things like what bloods to send off or what painkillers to prescribe. I don't think anyone has actually come to harm because we are quite a well-staffed department, luckily. I'm just worried about him when he's on his own and having to make decisions and just think that he might need a little bit more support.

**D:** It definitely sounds as though it's something we need to look into and maybe he is aware he is struggling himself and doesn't really know what to do.

Verbalising thoughts

**H:** Possibly.

**D:** It is very stressful starting as a new a doctor who has recently qualified but when you've been working for 6 months you should be able to deal with basic things, at least recognising unwell patients and knowing when to call for help.

**H:** Yes, quite and I think that's what I'm most worried about.

**D:** Have you or anyone else spoken to him directly yet?

**H:** I did tell him that day that I was worried about the patient and he should have called his senior.

**D:** OK. And how did he respond?

**H:** He apologised and said he was a bit nervous and flustered.

**D:** OK, so just to summarise. You are worried that Dr Peters is not really coping at the moment. He doesn't seem to handle the pressure well and seems to lack the confidence and ability to deal with straightforward problems. You aren't aware of any serious incidents occurring as a result but clearly this is a risk.

Summarising

**H:** That's right.

**D:** I really think it would be worth speaking to him about the situation and finding out things from his perspective in terms of how he feels that he's doing. It's important that he feels supported and not victimised. He may be finding his on calls very stressful and could need a lot more support and education. It is also possible that there are some outside stresses affecting his work performance.

Demonstrating compassion and empathy

**H:** Yes, that's a good point.

**D:** I think I should also speak to his educational supervisor to find out if any concerns have been raised about him by anyone else through any of his 360° appraisals and so that a plan can be made to ensure that he is performing safely and with enough support. Do you think this is a good idea?

Checking colleague agrees with plan

**H:** Yes, I think that would be important because I can imagine that other people have noticed this as well as myself, especially people who are working closely with him.

**D:** I can't really say what will happen from now on. I will have to leave these decisions to his clinical and educational supervisor but if you have any concerns about any patients then please feel free to bleep me, or one of my colleagues, and we would, of course, be happy to review.

Being open and honest
Remaining accessible to contact

**H:** Thank you – that's great.

## Healthcare professional scenario 9

| Transcript | Skills demonstrated |
|---|---|
| **D:** Hello Julie, do come in. | Used colleague's name |
| **H:** Thank you | |
| **D:** How are you? | Open question |
| **H:** I'm OK. Thank you for seeing me. I really just wanted to have a word with you about a couple of things. | |
| **D:** Of course, what did you want to talk about? | Open question |
| **H:** I just wanted to talk about my father who's been quite unwell recently. He's been diagnosed with bowel cancer. It's just really weird because I am so used to this sort of thing as I work here in a hospital, but I am just so shocked by it all. | |
| **D:** I'm sorry to hear that. What has happened to date? | Empathy |
| **H:** He was diagnosed 4 weeks ago and he is still in hospital after surgery. I think he's been told to have chemotherapy now. I'm so worried about it as he looks so frail at the moment. He's just become so weak and I don't know if he's going to be able to manage the chemo now. | |
| **D:** That must be very hard for you to see. Have you spoken to the doctors in the hospital where he's being treated about what's going to happen now? | Empathy |
| **H:** Sort of. They said it hasn't spread anywhere, so that's quite good. | |
| **D:** Yes it is, very good. [*Pause.*] How are you coping? | |
| **H:** I am doing OK, I think. I'm trying to hold it together for my family. My mum's really stressed. She's got problems of her own with anxiety and has been over-reacting somewhat. I'm worried about her as well. She just thinks he's dying. My brother is in Australia and calls me everyday to find out what's going on. And then there's my daughter, who is really struggling. She has been so close to her grandad as she stays with my parents when I am on shifts. | |
| **D:** It does sound as though you've got a huge amount going on – how are things affecting you? | Empathy |

**H:** I'm worried and anxious about it all and have a lot of pressure with Sophie at the moment as my mum can't really cope with looking after her without my dad around. I'm not really sleeping as well as I keep worrying about everything.

**D:** How old is your daughter?

**H:** She's 8.

**D:** Have you got any other support networks around you?

**H:** Yes, I've got a few close friends who have been really great and they are helping me with collecting Sophie from school when I'm working late but I don't want to put anyone out for too long. I'm sure they don't mind at the moment but it can't really be permanent.

**D:** And how are things at work for you?

**H:** Yes, that's one of the worst things. I keep seeing patients who are dying and when I go visit my father I keep thinking the worst and thinking of all the relatives I have seen coming to see their dying parents.

**D:** I know, working in these situations can be very hard. Have you spoken to any of the other nurses or the ward sister about it?

**H:** No, not really. I suppose I could try. I just don't really want to make a big thing about it and talk about it too much.

**D:** Have you thought about taking a little bit of time off if you're feeling so stressed and things are so difficult at home with childcare?

**H:** I would ideally like to but I had a slipped disc in my back last year and ended up taking about 4 weeks off. I just don't want people to think that I'm taking liberties and most of all I don't want to lose my job over it.

**D:** I do understand this is very difficult. Is there anything in particular you feel that I could help you with?

Exploring psychosocial factors and impact on work

Empathy

Reflecting back and problem solving

Exploring expectations

H: I don't really know. I just thought I don't have much experience of this and I just don't know if it is worth taking time off or what I should do.

D: Well, it's important to reflect upon how you're managing and coping with work. If you feel that your work is being affected it may be worth at least telling others around you what is going on so they can be a bit more understanding. If there are things you need help with you can also ask. I think it would be quite a good idea if you spoke to some of the nursing staff just to let them know what is going on. The other thing that you could do is to see your own GP about all the stress and the fact that you're not sleeping very well. I'm sure they will be able to offer you some help and advice.

*Demonstrating understanding and suggesting solutions to the problem*

H: That would be something I suppose, I never really thought about going to my GP.

D: There are also people such as myself around the wards if ever you are finding it really difficult and want to talk. If you did need to take some sort of compassionate leave, I am sure your line manager would understand and I really don't think you should fear losing your job. You are trying to cope with a huge amount and we should understand.

*Offering support*

H: Yes, I might do.

D: Going back to your family, especially regarding your brother who is calling you for advice. It seems to me that you are feeling a lot of pressure because of this.

*Reflecting back*

H: Definitely.

D: This is just a suggestion but it may be worth having a word with your brother and asking him to speak directly to the medical team as they would be able to give him more of an idea of what's going on with your father.

H: I know. I should do that.

D: You also mentioned that your mother is struggling with anxiety – maybe she should be encouraged to see her GP.

*Reflecting back*

H: Yes, I'll try to persuade her.

| | |
|---|---|
| **D:** I'm very happy that you have talked to me. Would it be OK if we touch base in the next few days to see how things are going and find out what you decide to do in terms of work? | Organising follow-up |
| **H:** That would be great – thank you so much for talking to me about this. | |
| **D:** If there's anything else you want to talk to me about just come and find me. I sincerely hope that your father is OK. | Sensitivity |
| **H:** Thanks. | |

## Healthcare professional scenario 10

| Transcript | Skills demonstrated |
|---|---|
| **D:** Hello Kim, come on in. | Used colleague's name |
| **H:** Hi there Dr Jacobs. Would it be okay if I just spoke to you for a couple of minutes? | |
| **D:** Of course. How can I help? | Open questions |
| **H:** Well, you are mess president aren't you? | |
| **D:** Yes, that's right. | |
| **H:** I'm absolutely fed up and I've just had enough! | |
| **D:** I am sorry to hear that – what has been going on? | Empathy |
| **H:** I have been cleaning this mess for a long time and that's exactly what it is – a complete and utter mess. My job is to clean but not tidy up after everyone. I have to wash your cups and plates, remove banana skins from the floor – it is getting ridiculous. | |
| **D:** I'm sorry things have been going wrong and I can understand why you are so angry about this. | Empathy<br>Acknowledging emotion |
| **H:** Well, wouldn't you be? | |
| **D:** Yes, I probably would. | |

**H:** It is an absolute disgrace and I cannot believe the lack of respect that you doctors are showing. I used to be able to clean this place in an hour but this is now taking me 3 hours a day and I'm just not prepared to do this anymore. I have other places in this hospital to clean and there is nowhere else where I feel so annoyed at the level of dirt and untidiness!

**D:** You are right, you shouldn't be tidying up after everyone and I am sorry it has got to this stage. Have you thought about how we can tackle this problem?

Empathy
Dealing with anger
Exploring ideas

**H:** No, not really. Any attempts that I have made have just failed and made me feel worse.

**D:** What sort of things have you tried?

Picking up on cue

**H:** Well, the other day I put a note up in the kitchen asking everyone to clean up after themselves and wash their cups and do you know what somebody had the nerve to write? 'Do it yourself'! Can you believe that? When I saw that I was absolutely livid because, at the end of the day, you may be doctors but we are all human beings and you have a responsibility to at least put your own rubbish in the bin.

**D:** I'm really sorry that this has happened and I'm so sorry that somebody wrote that on your note. I completely agree that that was rude and entirely unacceptable. As mess president I will take responsibility for ensuring that the situation improves. I'm really pleased that you've brought this to my attention. How long do you feel this has been a problem for?

Taking responsibility and apologising

**H:** For at least 4 or 5 months.

**D:** Well now that I know what's been going on I can try and do my best to improve things for you. Do you have any thoughts about what I could do?

Exploring ideas and expectations

**H:** Yes, I want you to tell everybody that they need to clean up after themselves and anybody that doesn't will have to face some serious consequences.

**D:** And I quite agree that people should be tidying up after themselves and definitely not leaving cups unwashed and banana skins on the floor. I'm happy to tell everybody that I can what's going on and it may be worth circulating an e-mail to all the junior doctors to tell them this has become a problem, just to increase awareness. How do you feel about that?

Checking agreement with plan

**H:** Yes, that would be great but I also want you to keep an eye out for people who are leaving things and tell them as they doing it, as I don't believe that things are going to change very quickly unless someone is actively monitoring what's going on.

**D:** I'm happy to do that as well. Sometimes with these situations things spiral out of control, people see others leaving their cups on the table and follow suit. I need to change behaviour and make sure that everyone realises the rules. I don't want you to have to wash everything up for us so it may even be worth leaving dirty cups unwashed on the side.

**H:** Well, that's pretty difficult because if I don't look like I'm doing my job and the mess is dirty I'll just get in trouble with my line manager. This is already happening as I'm not able to get round to cleaning other departments that I've been allocated because of the time I'm spending in the mess.

**D:** Have you been able to speak to your line manager about the problems you've had with the mess and the fact that it's taking you longer because it's so untidy?

Picking up on cue

**H:** I've tried that and it's not really helped. I have a lot of pressure on me at the moment and I really can't afford to annoy my line manager as I'll just end up losing my job.

**D:** Is that something you are worried about?

Picking up on cue

**H:** Well yes, my husband has been made redundant and I know the NHS is making cutbacks so it would be a disaster if I also got sacked. I've been staying later to make sure all of my work is done so my manager has no excuses to sack me.

**D:** I am sorry to hear about your husband. It must be a very stressful time for you and staying late at work can't help. How is it affecting you at home?

Exploring impact on home life

**H:** Well it was my husband who told me to speak to you. He is a bit fed up with me ranting and raving at home!

**D:** Well I hope if I can intervene and make things better here, then hopefully you won't feel you're under so much pressure. Would it help if I spoke to your line manager?

Offering solutions

**H:** No, I think if you could just try and get your colleagues to clean up after themselves I'd be more than happy and hopefully that way I can just leave on time, get my work done and not be so annoyed every time I come in here.

**D:** That's definitely something I'm going to do and I'll be keeping my eye out to be more vigilant about things around me. I'll also tell a few of the others who are involved with the mess on the committee to keep an eye on things. After I've managed to send out an e-mail and speak to some of the other doctors here, would it be possible if I meet with you in the next couple of weeks to see if you've noticed an improvement?

Organising follow-up

**H:** Yes, that would be quite useful.

**D:** And of course if it hasn't then I'll definitely need to escalate this further, possibly to some of the senior consultants so they can also become involved. It may end up being that our rights to drink tea and coffee and eat in the mess have to be temporarily removed if people are not tidying up.

**H:** Thanks for being so understanding and I do appreciate you apologising as well.

**D:** I'm sorry again about all of this and I'll see you in the next couple of weeks.

**H:** Thanks.

# Healthcare professional scenario 11

| Transcript | Skills demonstrated |
|---|---|
| **D:** Hello Mr Yates, come on in. | Used colleague's name |
| **H:** Hi Dr Newton. Thanks for seeing me. | |
| **D:** That's no problem at all. How can I help? | Open question |
| **H:** I just wanted to have a word about some of the doctors and also a few things that I've been seeing that's happening around the wards. As you may be aware, I'm the lead infection control nurse, which obviously makes me highly unpopular with you doctors! But I'm really just a little frustrated about the fact that a lot of the guidance for infection control is being ignored. | |
| **D:** Would you tell me little bit more about that? | Open question |
| **H:** Well yes. I mean, we have clear policies now about basic things such as being bare below the elbows, no watches, no jewellery, hair being tied back and hand washing, and I spend most of my days wandering around having to tell members of staff to adhere to these simple rules. | |
| **D:** Do have you any thoughts as to why staff won't adhere to the rules? | Exploring ideas |
| **H:** I've got no idea. I suppose they think it doesn't make any difference and it's just me nagging them. That's what it seems like from the way they pull faces at me. | |
| **D:** What do you mean? Have people been rude to you? | Active listening – responding to what your colleague said by picking up on cue |
| **H:** People have been making faces behind my back and laughing at me! I think the general attitude of the junior doctors is really quite bad. I don't enjoy telling people off but this is a very serious issue. I told an FY2 doctor that she needed to roll up her sleeves the other day and I saw her 5 minutes later and she had pulled them down again. I just cannot understand what is going on. | |
| **D:** I understand why this must be so frustrating for you. You are trying to act in the patients' best interests and not only are you feeling unsupported, but staff have been rude. That is completely unacceptable and I'm sorry you have experienced that. | Empathy<br><br>Encouraging |

**H:** It's also a little bit worrying because there are reasons that we ask people to do this. I don't thing it's a co-incidence that we have a bad reputation for infection rates. There has been an MRSA outbreak on the surgical wards recently and last year three wards were closed with a *Clostridium difficile* outbreak. I keep getting called in to speak to the managers to explain the high infection rates. I think they are losing patience with me.

**D:** That must be very stressful for you.

Empathy

**H:** Yes – many more outbreaks of infection and I think they'll get rid of me.

**D:** Is that something you are very worried about?

Picking up on cue

**H:** Well, I have been here for years so I think I've got a bit of goodwill and I don't think it will come to that.

**D:** I am really glad you have raised this issue. We all have responsibility to adhere to infection control rules and procedures. Did you have any thoughts about what we could do to improve the situation?

Exploring ideas and expectations

**H:** I just wanted to talk to somebody about this and thought you may be able to talk with the rest of your colleagues. And if you have any ideas of what we could do that would also be quite useful as I've tried going around and telling people off and being on patrol the whole time, and it doesn't seem to be working.

**D:** I think we need to increase awareness of this problem and of infection control rates. Have there been any audits carried out on hand washing or general infection rates on wards?

Problem solving

**H:** Oh yes, we have a record of the wards that need to be shut down and we are in the process of auditing hand washing and hygiene as well.

**D:** I would be very interested to know these results and this is a way that we can actually present some information at one of our clinical meetings, in order to try and increase awareness of the problem. I do think it's important to reiterate to all staff what the rules are about being bare below the elbow. It may be worth telling the nursing staff to keep an eye out and ask doctors who aren't adhering to this to sort it out. This might take the pressure off you a little bit as well so you can do other things.

Coming up with sensible solution

**H:** That would be a good idea.

**D:** Have you had a discussion with anyone else about this, such as senior consultants or colleagues?

**H:** No, not really. I was thinking about doing that but I thought I'd try and sort it out with some juniors first. Sometimes I think consultants are probably the worst with their suits and cufflinks and ties!

**D:** You are probably right. Would you be happy for me to raise this issue at our next clinical meeting or I could also talk to my consultant to get some advice about how we could solve this problem?

Checking colleague happy with plan

**H:** Yes, that would be brilliant and that's exactly the sort of thing I was hoping you would say you would do.

**D:** It is important that we do something quickly, because if infection rates are high and there are ways in which we can reduce patients coming to harm in this way, then it is vital that we act quickly to minimise this. Is there anything else you are concerned about?

Acknowledging patient safety potentially at risk

**H:** The only other thing, and it probably isn't too much of my business, is the fact that some of the female staff are not only having their long hair down but also wearing quite inappropriate clothing for a hospital environment. I've seen girls wear short skirts and low-cut tops! This sort of thing used to be frowned upon previously and people used to be sent home to change. I think that there should be some sort of dress code or even uniform for doctors. It's just so inappropriate.

**D:** Well yes, I can see why that is entirely inappropriate in the workplace. I'm sure other people have noticed that as well. Maybe we should be making more of this sort of thing at the inductions to warn people they will be asked to change clothes if they are thought to be inappropriate.

**H:** Yes, that would be great if you could.

**D:** We have talked about quite a lot today so would you mind if I just recapped?

Signposting

**H:** Not at all.

| Transcript | Skills demonstrated |
|---|---|
| **D:** You have understandably been feeling under pressure trying to get staff, especially junior doctors, to adhere to the infection control rules. At times doctors have been rude to you despite you only trying to do your job. To try to help I have agreed to discuss this at one of our clinical meetings, when ideally I would be able to present some audit data to highlight this problem. There is also the issue of inappropriate clothing. I know this can be a tricky issue so it may be sensible to include guidelines in the induction pack. Is that OK? | Summarising |
| **H:** That's great, thanks. | |
| **D:** Can I arrange to see you again to look through some of the audit data and also discuss any other ideas that the consultants may have to help with this problem? | Organising follow-up |
| **H:** Yes, that's great. I'm away next week but I can meet you when I get back. | |
| **D:** OK. You've got my details so give me a call when you're back. Hopefully we'll get this sorted out as soon as possible. | |
| **H:** Thank you. | |
| **D:** Have a good holiday and I'll see when you get back. | |

# Healthcare professional scenario 12

| Transcript | Skills demonstrated |
|---|---|
| **D:** Hi Sophie, come in. | Used colleague's name |
| **D:** I understand you wanted to have a quick word? | Opening remark |
| **H:** Yes, thanks for taking the time to have a chat with me. | |
| **D:** What seems to be the problem? | Open question |
| **H:** I just wanted to talk to somebody in confidence about something. I'm really sorry if I've been a little bit short with people at the practice but it's just that I've been struggling for the last few weeks. | |
| **D:** Oh, what's been going on? | Open question |

H: Well at the moment I'm pregnant and it's been a really difficult time in the last few weeks, as I've just been feeling so ill.

D: How are you feeling about this pregnancy?

Clarifying feelings about the pregnancy

H: Oh, I'm really happy about it. I know I sound a bit down because I've been feeling ill, but this is amazing news for me and my husband. It's just that I've been so worried about the whole pregnancy and it's also been difficult for me with no one knowing. I'm only just about able to do my clinics and keep up to date with my work really.

D: Well, congratulations. Do you mind me asking how many weeks you are?

H: Yes, 10 weeks today actually.

D: You mentioned you were quite worried about it. Was there any particular reason for that?

Reflecting back and picking up on cue

H: Well, it's just that I didn't really want to tell anybody because it's still early days and we're really happy to be pregnant but so worried about things not working out.

D: Is there any particular reason you're worried about that?

H: I've had a bad experience in the past as we had a missed miscarriage. I told everyone when I was 6 weeks and it was just so awful having to tell everyone after. Now I've been trying to get pregnant for the last 3 years so this pregnancy is long overdue!

D: Gosh, I can see why it's been so worrying for you.

Empathy

H: Yes I know.

D: And in what way have you been feeling unwell?

Reflecting back

H: I have been absolutely shattered and feeling really sick all the time. I have had to vomit between my patients and it's just got to a point where I feel so unwell I'm struggling to keep to time. There are some mornings where I'm finding it difficult to get to work. I think people are noticing that I've not been doing as well as I normally do.

**D:** It can be very hard in early pregnancy. Has anyone said anything to you?

Empathy

**H:** One of the partners last week had a big go at me because I didn't do some paperwork that I was supposed to do.

**D:** Well, it definitely sounds like it's a really stressful time for you, not only because you feel physically sick, but also because you've understandably been worried about everything from past experiences. Have you discussed the pregnancy with anyone else at the practice yet?

Empathy

**H:** Not yet as I want to keep it quiet in case I was to have another miscarriage. I'd hate to have to tell everyone that it had gone wrong again.

**D:** I can understand that. Apart from not running to time and struggling to get in at 7 am, do you feel that your performance at work is otherwise okay?

**H:** Yes, it's fine and you know I'm just about managing clinics and I haven't made any clinical mistakes or anything like that. I just feel really sick.

**D:** And how are things at home for you?

**H:** Everything is fine. Obviously Jack, my husband, is also quite nervous about the whole situation. He's been great considering I've not been the best company to be around. He's quite busy with his work and he wants me to tell people here so that everyone understands why I've been off par.

**D:** Have you had any thoughts as to how you want to proceed from now?

Exploring ideas

**H:** Well no, not really. I just needed to tell someone at work it has been quite difficult for me to keep this to myself.

**D:** I do understand where you're coming from. You are 10 weeks pregnant now so the chance of having a miscarriage is small. It may be worth just telling the partners here so that they understand you are struggling and could make some easy changes. You could maybe start clinics later and have longer gaps between patients.

Making suggestions

**H:** That would be brilliant if they could do that but I just don't know how people react to me.

**D:** I know that you are worried about it but you will have to tell them at some point and I think everyone will be happy for you. The other thing to say is that I'm sure the GPs would be very sensitive towards you if something were to happen during the pregnancy, and it may be good to get some support, even if the worst case scenario were to happen.

**H:** Yes, I can see your point.

**D:** Was there anything you wanted me to do to help you?

**H:** Not really. I just wanted somebody to know what was going on.

**D:** And I'm really glad you've told me – congratulations again. How are you feeling at the moment?

**H:** Well, I'm OK. I've got another clinic this afternoon so I've got quite a bit to do today.

**D:** Well I'm always around as well so, if you are really struggling and you need a hand please just come and let me know. Would you prefer that I had a word with one of the partners or anyone else in practice?

**H:** No, that's fine. I think you're right, I should probably tell some of them because I wouldn't want them to think I am underperforming for any reason or think that there is something else going on with me.

**D:** I think you'll find people will be very supportive towards you. If you have any more problems please do just come in and let me know, or when you just want to chat. Have you seen your own GP about your sickness, as there are things that can be done for you that you can take for this?

**H:** No and I think I'm OK at the moment. I'd prefer not to take anything during this pregnancy and I'm sure it will get better.

**D:** OK. Well let me know how you get on talking to the partners and if there is anything else I can do, just ask.

**H:** Thank you very much.

| | |
|---|---|
| Reassurance | |
| Exploring expectations | |
| Offering support | |
| Reassuring colleague | |

# Healthcare professional scenario 13

| Transcript | Skills demonstrated |
|---|---|
| **D:** Hi Sue, come in. | Used colleague's name |
| **D:** How can I help? | Open question |
| **H:** I wanted to talk to you about something that's been bugging me. | |
| **D:** Of course. | |
| **H:** I saw Angie our health visitor take 10 quid out of the petty cash box last week. She thinks no one saw but she definitely did it when she was putting the temporary permit back in the drawer. | |
| **D:** Oh dear. Did you say anything at the time? | |
| **H:** I was so shocked I didn't know what to do. I suppose I should have just asked her what she was doing but I sort of panicked. | |
| **D:** Yes, I can imagine it was an awkward situation to find yourself in. Was anyone else there? | Empathy |
| **H:** No just me – but she definitely did it and it will probably be on the CCTV as well. | |
| **D:** OK, well this is a very tricky but important issue. Obviously trust and probity are very important issues for healthcare professionals. | Probity |
| **D:** Have you tried to discuss this with anyone else? | |
| **H:** No. I thought about telling the practice manager but I really don't want to talk to him right now. I can barely stand to be in the same room as that man, let alone talk to him! | |
| **D:** Do you mind me asking why that is? | Picking up on cue |
| **H:** He is just intolerable and awful. He has made me feel so bad lately and accused me of messing up the appointments a few weeks ago when he put on clinics that he shouldn't have. I mean, that is the main part of his job and he cannot | |

admit when he messes things up. He had the nerve to then tell the partners at their meeting that I was being rude to patients. I have been here long enough for the doctors to know what I'm like so luckily they agreed I had done nothing wrong. Since then Keith is just so rude to me. He just gives me nasty looks and ignores me now.

**D:** Oh dear, that sounds like it has been very difficult for you lately.

Empathy

**H:** Yes, so you can imagine why I don't want Angie hating me too.

**D:** I see. Did you have any thoughts as to what would could be done from here

Exploring ideas and expectations

**H:** Not really, I thought of challenging her but what would I say? 'Oh Angie, why did you steal £10?' She would just deny it and then I'd have another enemy.

**D:** You are right – it would be very hard. I think we need to consider this carefully. It is important to get to the bottom of the issue. Just thinking out loud, there may be an explanation – perhaps she was owed the £10, or she had maybe left it as a deposit for the permit. I don't know but she certainly needs a chance to explain herself. It's probably also worth looking at the CCTV as you say. I'm not entirely sure how to approach this and think you should discuss this with the partners. How do you feel about that?

Discussing plans

Verbalising thoughts
Being honest about not knowing exactly what to do

**H:** I think that's probably a good idea. I'll try and talk to Dr Sams tomorrow.

**D:** Do you have any other worries about Angie with regard to this sort of thing or her work?

**H:** No, she is really quite sweet and I've always got on with her really well. She has never talked about being hard up or anything.

**D:** The other thing you talked about before was your relationship with Keith. It sounds as though things have been, and continue to be, quite strained between you?

**H:** Oh yeah. He's such a difficult person. It's not only me though, we all think he's awful.

**D:** This is a very important issue. It's not right that staff don't trust the practice manager and I think you should probably explain the situation to Dr Sams. It certainly sounds as though something needs to be done because it is not a good atmosphere to be working in at the moment.

Reflecting back

**H:** You are right there – I used to love work but now I dread coming in.

**D:** That is such a shame and something clearly needs to be done. How is it affecting you?

**H:** I'm a bit down about it but I'm hopeful things will get better.

**D:** Thank you for speaking to me about this, it must have been stressful coping with it alone. Perhaps we could speak again once you have spoken to Dr Sams, just to make sure everything is sorted out.

Organising follow-up

**H:** Thank you, that would be good.

## Healthcare professional scenario 14

| Transcript | Skills demonstrated |
|---|---|
| **D:** Good afternoon Rebecca, come in. | Used colleague's name |
| **H:** Hi, thank you for speaking to me. | |
| **D:** How are you? | Open question |
| **H:** I'm stressed – I'm so stupid and I just wanted to tell someone what I've done. | |
| **D:** OK, what's that? | Open question |
| **H:** I am going to be in so much trouble! I can't believe how stupid I am sometimes. If anyone's seen what I've said I'm going to get in so much trouble! | |
| **D:** You seem very stressed. Can I ask you what you think you may be in trouble about? | Acknowledging emotion |

H: Oh sorry. I'm in a bit of a state because I went to the lunchtime meeting today and the chief executive was talking about taking disciplinary action against staff making comments about anything related to the hospital on social networking sites. I had no idea and I've already said so much!

D: Oh right, I see.

H: I mean, I updated my online status yesterday. What do you think will happen?

D: I don't know exactly what was said at the meeting today but what sort of things have you been writing online?

*Clarifying details of the problem*

H: Just stuff. Sometimes it's just things like 'I can't be bothered to go into work today', but sometimes I've been saying stuff about the nursing staff and how I think the care here is really bad for patients. It's really bad now I think about it and I totally realise I am in the wrong. It's so unprofessional.

D: OK. Well I am pleased you have come to talk to me about this. I can see it is really worrying you. I do agree with what you said about it being unprofessional to write things in the public domain about work, but the main thing now is that it's been brought to your attention and I suspect you won't do it again.

H: Oh my goodness, never again.

D: How long have you been writing things related to work on this website for?

H: I don't know. It's not often but when I get frustrated I tend to express it online. I suppose it has been for the past few years.

D: I must say this is something I've never really come across before, but I imagine you aren't alone in writing things like this. I suspect this is why it was mentioned at the meeting. Have you had any thoughts about what to do now?

*Exploring ideas (what is your colleague thinking they should do)*

H: Well, I have deleted everything and changed my privacy settings so that now only friends can see my photos and posts, but the managers said that they had already seen some examples and would be following these up.

**D:** Lots of people seem to fall into the trap of thinking these social networking sites are private when in fact they are quite the opposite. Well done for taking all of the comments down. I suppose you have a couple of options: you could contact your managers and advise them that in the past you have made comments about work or you could hope that your comments were not seen by anyone and that no damage has been done. What are your thoughts?

**H:** Oh no, I don't think I could tell my managers – then I would definitely be in trouble. That would mean they would probably have a look and then I'll get in so much trouble.

**D:** Can you to give me an example of the sort of things you have been posting?

**H:** I have said something along the lines of the fact that I can't stand to sit around watching the nurses while they ignore the poor elderly patients who are shouting for help.

**D:** Yes, you mentioned before that you thought the care here was really bad. Is this something you believe is happening on the wards on a regular basis?

Reflecting back – showing you have been listening
Picking up on cues

**H:** Oh completely. They are really awful, especially on the care of the elderly ward I'm working on at the moment. That doesn't make me saying it on a social networking site any more acceptable though.

**D:** No it doesn't, but you are raising very important issues. Have you thought about discussing your concerns with the ward sister? It doesn't sound like something that can be ignored, especially if you believe patients are being neglected and may be coming to harm.

Ensuring patient safety paramount concern

**H:** I've been thinking about this for a while and I think that I should. It really upsets me seeing patients not being cared for correctly. It is the same everywhere – I saw it in Manchester when my mother was in hospital as well, and I had a patient's son complaining to me the other day about the same thing and I didn't know what to say. Maybe I should speak to one of the senior sisters about it.

| | |
|---|---|
| **D:** I agree. It's something that can't really be ignored. I think there are wards that are fantastically well run with incredibly dedicated nurses but sometimes, for various reasons, the quality of care on other wards may suffer and this needs to be looked into. I'm really pleased you have brought all of this up today and I hope you are feeling less stressed. Can you run through what you're going to do from now on? | Giving a balanced view |
| **H:** Well, I've already deleted everything and obviously I'll never do it again. I think I'll also try and have a word with the senior sister on the ward about my concerns as well. | |
| **D:** That sounds like a very sensible plan. Would you like to arrange a time to see me again about this to discuss this further? | Organising follow-up |
| **H:** I think I should be OK. I feel a lot calmer now. | |
| **D:** Well, I will be around and you have my bleep in case you do want to speak again. | |

## Healthcare professional scenario 15

| Transcript | Skills demonstrated |
|---|---|
| **D:** Hello Mrs Jones. Come in. | Used colleague's name |
| **H:** Oh, do call me Marilyn. | |
| **D:** Of course Marilyn, how can I help? | Open question |
| **H:** Yes. It's about Dr Hemley. I hate telling on someone and I was going to give him the benefit of the doubt but it's just one thing after another you know. Last night was the final straw. | |
| **D:** OK, what has been happening? | Open question |
| **H:** I know he comes across as a really enthusiastic doctor to all of you guys on the ward, but having been a ward clerk for over a decade, I have seen doctors like him before. He puts on a very keen front but actually seems to avoid work when he's on the ward and has been quite rude to me on a few occasions. I get worried about bleeping him for anything as a few months ago he shouted at me for calling him for some notes. | |

**D:** Thank you for speaking to me about this. There are some very important issues that you have raised. You also mentioned that last night was the final straw – can I ask what happened?

Picking up on cues

**H:** Well, you may be aware he's been off sick this week. He's been ringing me every morning, but last night I was out and I saw him at the cinema with his friends. I couldn't believe it – he had clearly been drinking as well.

**D:** That is not at all fair.

**H:** I know. He then called me today to say he was still sick. I wanted to tell him I saw him out last night but I didn't in the end.

**D:** You also said that he had been rude to you – that is not acceptable – what has happened?

**H:** Well, he is always cross; he answers the bleep rudely and is always reluctant to come. He seems to think we are all wasting his time.

**D:** I am sorry that you have had to experience that. Before we move on to talk about what ought to be done is there anything else that you have noticed?

Empathy
Signposting

**H:** No, that is it I think.

**D:** Thank you very much for bringing it up with me as it's so important that this sort of thing is raised for the benefit of the team, the patients and Dr Hemley himself as he needs to be aware of how to behave professionally. It is completely unacceptable to lie about sickness and to be rude to any member of staff at work. It sounds like it is a general attitude problem, but sometimes there are things happening inside or outside of work causing such frustration. It certainly needs to be looked into. Have you noticed any patients' care being affected as a result of his actions?

Ensuring patient care not affected

**H:** No – I think the team cover for him when he is away – but of course that is not fair on them.

**D:** Did you have any thoughts about what should be done?

Exploring ideas

**H:** I don't think I should have to challenge him. He will just ignore me.

**D:** I agree. I don't think you should have to deal with this yourself. I could certainly speak to him and if his behaviour doesn't improve dramatically then it is probably something that should be raised with his consultant or educational supervisor.

Problem solving

**H:** That would be good.

**D:** I will definitely have a chat with Dr Hemley about his general attitude and behaviour that you mentioned and about the fact that he has been calling in sick when he's been seen out.

**H:** That would be really good but I'd rather he didn't know it was me who has reported him.

**D:** OK, I don't think it would be a problem to keep you out of it this at this stage, but I suppose the consultant may wish to speak to you if it is escalating.

**H:** OK, yes, I can understand that.

**D:** Could we possibly meet again in a few weeks to make sure that his performance has improved?

Organising follow-up

**H:** Yes of course. That would be good.

**D:** Just to mention, if you do feel Dr Hemley is rude to you or does anything else in the meantime, please do come and let myself or one of the team know.

**H:** I will. Thanks.